PRAISE FOR

All That Moves Us

One of the Best Books of the Year:
The New Yorker, Publishers Weekly

"Vivid . . . [Jay Wellons's] book unfolds in a harrowing series of operating-room vignettes, explaining the work of his hands while also evoking the tension in his mind and his heart. . . . Identifying this drive to narrate—to tell stories as a human once the doctor's work is done—is perhaps the key insight of Wellons's book." —*The New Yorker*

"A powerful and moving account of the intense joys and sorrows of being a pediatric neurosurgeon."

—Henry Marsh, *New York Times* bestselling author of
Do No Harm: Stories of Life, Death, and Brain Surgery

"As a surgeon, Jay Wellons has long healed with his hands. What this engaging and illuminating book shows us is how important the heart is in the life and work of a doctor charged with the sacred—even staggering—task of operating on the brains of children. At once reflective and searching, Wellons's stories from the journey give us hope that light can emerge from even the darkest of hours."

—Jon Meacham, #1 *New York Times* bestselling author of
His Truth Is Marching On: John Lewis and the Power of Hope

"Reading *All That Moves Us* feels like watching a full season of your favorite medical drama, complete with harrowing surgical scenes and meaningful reflections within each episode. In bearing witness to some of life's most profound moments, Jay Wellons has written an extraordinarily memorable book." —Mary Laura Philpott, author of
Bomb Shelter: Love, Time, and Other Explosives

Healing Together

―――・◦・―――

A Note on the Paperback Cover

JAY WELLONS

S URGERY IS SCARY at any age, but particularly for children. They don't want to be separated from Mom and Dad. They don't want to be with total strangers rolling down a hall on a gurney into a bright room marked STERILE on the door. And they sure don't want to be lying on a bed in the center of that bright room with unfamiliar masked people milling around them, going back and forth to computer screens or instrument trays. Oh, everyone greets them kindly when they arrive, particularly the OR nurses—a special group of people, with a smile that can be seen around the edges of the mask and their kind eyes gleaming. Our anesthesia colleagues do their best to distract and comfort, too. The kids get to choose what flavor they can smell in the inhaled anesthetic mask. (Strawberry is popular. Banana is not.) Small talk about superheroes or their favorite toys or sports team mixes with the quiet chatter of the OR circulating nurse and scrub tech as they begin to carefully prepare the back scrub tables by laying out sterile blue drapes. I've watched all this play out thousands of times from the side of the room, where we, as the surgical team, sit and await the word from the anesthesiologist that we may move ahead with positioning and prepping, and the surgical procedure itself. But it is what the nurses do after the child goes to sleep that is my absolute favorite. And that's where the new cover for this book comes in.

Nearly without fail, the younger kids will be clutching a beloved stuffed animal as they make the journey into the operating room. Teddy bears, smiling foxes, purple elephants, toothy dinosaurs— I've seen all sorts of stuffed animals on that gurney over the years. I remember a plush scorpion (named Justin) next to a little boy as he fell off to sleep as we prepared to take out a sizable brain tumor that was giving him headaches. After all the instruments are laid out and verified and the checklists completed, it is finally time to start the actual operation. That's when the OR nurses get to work on the stuffed animals, stealing precious minutes during a break to carefully wrap the child's stuffed animal in its own surgical dressing, to match the dressing that the child will find themselves wrapped in when they wake up. And yes, the scorpion was fitted with a nifty headwrap. When its owner woke up and opened his eyes and became aware of his surroundings in the pediatric ICU, there was his best buddy, Justin, looking the same way. The child and the stuffed animal then heal together: In the days after surgery, when it is time for the headwrap to come off, off comes the headwrap on the stuffed animal as well. *Better be careful of that stinger, doctor.* IV removal time? The same for the animal. It's a kind and simple way to help a child understand what they are going through and that they are not alone. And isn't that really what helps most of all? Love, kindness, and healing . . . together. Like I said, it takes a special person to be a nurse in the pediatric OR.

Credit for cover bear: Kayla Grace Gross, RN, and Laura Newsom, CST

Photo credit: Edwin Tse Photography

All That Moves Us

ALL THAT
MOVES US

A Pediatric Neurosurgeon, His Young Patients,

and Their Stories of Grace and Resilience

———

JAY WELLONS

RANDOM HOUSE

New York

2023 Random House Trade Paperback Edition

Copyright © 2022 by John C. Wellons III, MD

Published in the United States by Random House, an imprint and division of Penguin Random House LLC, New York.

RANDOM HOUSE and the HOUSE colophon are registered trademarks of Penguin Random House LLC.

Originally published in hardcover in the United States by Random House, an imprint and division of Penguin Random House LLC, in 2022.

Library of Congress Cataloging-in-Publication Data
Names: Wellons, Jay, author.
Title: All that moves us: A pediatric neurosurgeon, his young patients, and their stories of grace and resilience / Jay Wellons.
Description: First edition. | New York: Random House, [2022] | Includes index.
Identifiers: LCCN 2021045920 (print) | LCCN 2021045921 (ebook) | ISBN 9780593243381 (trade paperback) | ISBN 9780593243374 (ebook)
Subjects: MESH: Central Nervous System Diseases—surgery | Child | Infant | Adolescent | Neurosurgical Procedures | Neurosurgeons | Pediatrics | Tennessee | Personal Narrative
Classification: LCC RD593 (print) | LCC RD593 (ebook) | NLM WS 340.5 | DDC 617.4/8083—dc23
LC record available at https://lccn.loc.gov/2021045920
LC ebook record available at https://lccn.loc.gov/2021045921

Printed in the United States of America on acid-free paper

randomhousebooks.com

2 4 6 8 9 7 5 3 1

To Melissa, Jack, and Fair; and to Mom and Dad

His soul swooned slowly as he heard the snow falling faintly through the universe and faintly falling, like the descent of their last end, upon all the living and the dead.

—James Joyce, "The Dead," *Dubliners*

Contents

Author's Note

THE STORIES IN *All That Moves Us* are true. The children, their parents, and my colleagues written about in these pages are real people. I spoke with nearly all the parents (or the patients themselves) in order to ensure that they would allow me to share the details of their respective journeys. I also sent the most recent version of the essay in which they or their child were mentioned. Each and every person that I communicated with gave me permission to use their child's (and/or their own) name and identifying information. In a few circumstances, I had the honor of reading the story to the parent in person and sharing the emotion relived, just for a moment.

There are some examples where I was unable to locate a parent, or a patient was not able to be found, and in those cases I did make changes to identifying characteristics to protect privacy. Some of my past co-worker names, such as in the chapter entitled "A Mississippi Nick," have also been altered. In all of these circumstances, none of the changes materially affected the reality of the lived experience.

Prologue

———•◦•———

The Littlest Among Us

I AM A PEDIATRIC neurosurgeon. That means I operate on children of all ages with brain and spinal cord problems. Those problems translate to tumors, blood vessel malformations, brain or skull development problems that need surgery, hydrocephalus, spina bifida, trauma; the list is long. I sew nerves back together if they are torn during birth using suture as fine as human hair. Some operations we do on teenagers on the verge of adulthood and some in the first week of life, including premature infants that weigh even less than one kilogram. I used to think that was small until I started doing spinal cord surgery on fetuses inside the uterus a few years back.

For the record, I don't usually lead at parties with my work. When people outside the hospital ask me what I do, I tell them I work in healthcare. Then, over about five more questions, if they take it that far, the term "pediatric neurosurgeon" finally comes out. My wife tells me that nothing can bring a party to a halt like talking about the importance of car seats and bicycle helmets, especially if I start telling stories from work.

My father had wanted to be a doctor. I feel it is important that you know that before we get started. Well before I was born, he had considered leaving a successful career in business and entering medical school. It was risky, but as a Korean War–era National Guard pilot he was used to risk. Earlier in his life, just after air force flight school and before the start of his first job, he had worked with a family medicine doctor, and the experience never left him. The kind older doctor had given my father his own stethoscope after their time together and told him that he would make a wonderful doctor one day. I have that stethoscope now. There is a little inscription on the bell that has Dad's name and "MD" after it. It's like a relic from an alternate history. In a brief one-year push after leaving the working world, my father took postgraduate classes and passed entrance tests and came to the very cusp of getting himself there, but by then he had two small children and a wife at home and no way to pay for it or to make any kind of living for them. He tried. I've seen the letters detailing unsuccessful attempts to secure the finances necessary for tuition. So, over time, he set that dream aside. Then, years later, I was born, a third child, very unexpected. From nearly that moment on, it was his hope that I would be a doctor.

At least initially, I fully bought into that dream. As a child, a few times I found myself interested in other careers. I was fascinated by flight and wore my father's flight helmet around the house. Taking that path, I was told, meant too much time away from family. *Such irony now.* Focus on what could be accomplished on the ground. I realized just how pleased my parents were when I wrote my grade school career essay on being a doctor.

Over time, like most teenagers and proto-adults, I decided to take a different path, *make my own way.* I became an English major and tried to focus on writing but somehow, *somehow* kept taking premed classes and did well enough on the MCAT to get into medical school. I studied Joyce and Yeats and Shakespeare in college with professors who had trained at Trinity College in Dublin and at Oxford, and I took creative writing from Barry Hannah one semester and Ellen Douglas the next. The former pinched the filters off whatever cigarettes he was chain-smoking at the time in our small by-permission-only class and gave me a B minus on my writing. The latter sat with me and helped me and later wrote to me in a copy of *Black Cloud, White Cloud,* "To Jay, whose works I remember with great fondness." (And no one knows until right now that I turned in the same stories to them both.) Despite all of that, I looked up after boarding school and college and found myself in medical school living my father's dream, and that was just fine. I thought maybe I was there to learn something about what it means to be alive. I really had no idea what was to unfold over the next twenty-five years.

I cannot even begin to count the number of people outside the field who told me *not* to be a neurosurgeon. *You are nothing like them,* they said. *Neurosurgeons are tired and grumpy. Egotistical. They work too much. The patients do terrible. Everyone dies.* At first, during my medicine rotation, I really liked cardiology. Listening to the heart and performing the physical exam became the hinge point on which all later decisions were based. Measured presentations, well-conceived plans. Did you know that you can diagnose aortic regurgitation by a bobbing uvula? Does anyone know that now? But back then we did. The men wore ties and the women wore scarves, and we slung our stethoscopes around our necks and diagnosed murmurs, rubs, gallops, squeaks, and rumbles as if we ruled each and every hall of the hospital. John Stone, the writer/cardiologist from Emory, had signed his book of essays for me when I was a first-year student and working in the cadaver lab. He said I smelled like formaldehyde. "To Jay, at the beginning . . ."

Three months later and I thought general pediatrics was terrific. The chief resident caught me coming in early one morning to feed the babies. *If you feed the babies, you're gonna do peds,* he said. But it wasn't *all* the babies. It was this one baby. He was by himself in the crib, no visitors ever. Born with an addiction to crack, I think. He was through the worst of it, but he was still alone. Other babies had family members come in every day, sit with them in rocking chairs. But not this one. I remember, even now, holding him in my lap early in the morning before anyone else would see me and looking down at his tiny head, the little ridge running down the middle where the bones overlapped under the skin. I would come in early to feed him and to try to let him feel what it was like to be safe. I just knew that I had so much love and support in my life to spare that it overflowed all around me, and I wanted him to feel just a little. But then after a few weeks, he was gone—discharged to where and with whom I was never told—and then I moved on to the next rotation, which was surgery.

Which is where I learned that I would *definitely* have to do something with my hands. I would stay and stay and stay, just to operate. I remember an attending named Dr. Reggie at the VA hospital during my third year as a medical student. Dr. Reggie would let me operate with him. *Let's see if Wellons was paying attention,* he would say to his resident. *Let him try those bowel stitches.* And I was. So I did. Late one night, we saved a vet from renal failure by cutting off his leg, which was dying and knocking out his one good kidney. The complicating issue was that there was a metal bar in his femur because of an old fracture, and we couldn't cut through it with the equipment we had in the OR at 2:00 in the morning. The electric blade was nearly vibrating me apart. So Dr. Reggie had the guys who work downstairs in maintenance help. They loved Dr. Reggie because he always treated them with respect. So he called them up into the OR in the middle of the night and asked them to find us the biggest saw they could and to sharpen it up and sterilize it while we waited. After a while, in was brought something you see contestants use in those two-person log-cutting contests. He and I went back and forth, back and forth, back and forth. There were sparks, I remember. The patient had to be awake but numbed under spinal anesthesia because he was too sick to go all the way under, the anesthesiologist concerned his blood pressure was too low and his heart couldn't take it. I remember him looking over at me, from around the drapes as I was sawing, and he said, "Lord Almighty." Then we were through it and my hands hurt but we saved him. I knew then that I wanted to save people.

Later, during my official surgery rotation, there was a pediatric general surgeon, Dr. Miller, who was beanpole tall and skinny, had *alopecia totalis,* no hair anywhere (they said), and was the busiest man I knew. He could do just about anything in the operating room. He had pulled more than a thousand coins out of kids' airways and stomachs, and he saved each coin in one of those little books with the slots. (I still have one of those books from my own childhood, full of coins in paper coin holders with clear plastic windows.) Over time, Dr. Miller cataloged the coins he had pulled out and figured out which coin was the most commonly swallowed. *Avoid those from the Denver Mint, I tell you.* He would regularly give a talk about how statistics could be misused to find a meaningless answer. He would teach us exam findings and X-ray reading every day on rounds and in the OR. Every Sunday morning he would put on a formal lecture to the students and residents he called Sunday school. He was beloved, and I wanted to teach as he did and be beloved by my students one day just as he was. His daughter was in my medical school class; I met her when I inadvertently flicked one of my cadaver's toenails into her grimy dissection coat pocket in the first month of class. Despite this, she became one of my closest friends, later a bridesmaid in my wedding. A few years ago, I left after my last patient in clinic one day to drive down to Mississippi to Dr. Miller's funeral. When I walked in, she, her husband, and their four teenage children all broke from the receiving line to hug my neck, and we all stood there and cried together for a while because *they* knew how much Dr. Miller meant to *me* and what he stood for and what he did for thousands and thousands of children. And for me.

So, from cardiology I knew I loved the physical exam and from pediatrics the innocents (note, not innocence). From surgery, I was drawn to working with my hands and saving people, and from Dr. Miller, I learned that I wanted to teach and be valued by my students one day. I knew it was time to decide on my residency, but I also knew that neurosurgeons were *burned out and not like me.*

But throughout my entire time in medical school, I would watch the sea of people part in the emergency department (ED) and in would come the neurosurgery resident. They would do a quick exam, order a CT, speak calmly with the families, then methodically move on to the next emergency. Walking down one problem after another. The ones I met were tired and grumpy and worked too much and acted a little odd with everyone else—me too, at first. It was like they lived in a different world from the rest. But pretty soon after I began a formal rotation with them, they didn't seem so odd anymore. They started teaching me about the brain and the spinal cord at any spare moment we could find. They would sit with me late into the night in the midst of the chaos of the ED around us and draw complex diagrams like the nerve innervation to the muscles of the arm or a rough drawing of the cranial nerves that I still draw for my students to this very day. The patients we took care of then had blood clots from car wrecks, spine injuries to fix, brain tumors we would take out, or all kinds of problems with their central nervous system that would take the patients, human beings just like you or me, nearly over the edge. And we would pull them back. Not always, but most of the time. I stayed at the hospital during Thanksgiving break of my third year of medical school just so I could work with the residents, and I remember feeling like I had two hands full of thumbs and was invincible at the same time.

For weeks, every time I would walk past the neurosurgery operating room, I would stop and look inside to see what they were doing. Not once or twice, but every time. *One hundred percent* of the time I would stand on my tiptoes to peek in through the little square window in the door. So, one day I decided that I would just see and I did see and I thought that I could connect with people and save people and teach people and be a neurosurgeon because I *was* like them in many ways, after all.

My first two years at Duke for my residency were a blur. That two-year blur turned into a six-year blur. How I had gotten to Duke

from Mississippi in the first place remains a mystery, but had something to do with the fact that when I rotated there for a month as
a medical student, I could work a long time without quitting, and
if I did not know an answer, I would not make something up but
would go find it out. The blurring of that time also comes from the
fact that in the last year of medical school, on the verge of my journey into this remarkable life to be lived, my father became ill with
ALS—amyotrophic lateral sclerosis—a relentless neurodegenerative disease leading to paralysis and death for which no surgery or
intervention is available. I left him in Mississippi, and one year later,
the busiest and most intense of my life to date, he was suddenly
gone and I was left with a path stretching out in front of me. For
all my uncertainty about how I would spend my life in medicine, it
is but one irony that I would devote my career to trying to better
understand the anatomical system that had failed my father. I know
now that I would come to see him in the patients that I cared for,
and also see myself in the families' grief.

The reality of life-and-death choices quickly burns away any idealized idea of invincibility. I remember early on an attending telling me he wanted my asshole to blanch when I took care of his
patients. He told me this while making a tight okay sign, his index
finger circled tightly within the crease of his thumb and squeezing it
tight enough to make the skin of the finger white—to be clear, the
whole thing representing my own anus, blanching. *Good gosh, where
am I?* I thought. We would work hours on end. I would fall asleep
with food in my mouth while eating. I hit the same tree—thankfully
on a slow curve—twice in a month while driving home well after
midnight. I fell asleep operating. No amount of caffeine or adrenaline can counter the kind of tired you get after being awake for two
nights straight on a routine basis. Now the term is "sleep deficit"
when fatigue builds up like that over time. Back then, it was just
how things were done, without question. You just persevered, or

you either dropped out or were fired. As a resident, you find quickly that you are just trying to stay afloat in the rapids without drowning until all of a sudden you are done.

Amid that chaos of becoming a neurosurgeon, I was drawn to the cases that involved children. I watched as the pediatric neurosurgeons moved with the parents and the children from the anxious unknown of diagnosis through the delicate surgical interventions and finally into the relief of recovery. For the child, it was simply a chance to heal and live; theirs is the most innocent view. *I hurt; now I hurt no longer.* For the parent, it was the intensity of the emotions that come with the anguish of a life-altering diagnosis in your child and the trust necessary to allow another human being to intervene. For the surgeon, it was the opportunity to fundamentally improve, or even bring back, a child who is pure potential, for whom nothing is truly determined and all possibilities exist.

There is a word, "pluripotent," typically used to describe stem cells, incredibly important microscopic structures within our bodies that have the ability to become nearly any other cell line—and this part is key—*depending on the influence.* Over the years of operating on child after child, often having a profound impact on their lives, feeling deeply blessed in order to have done so, and seeing them grow into adults, I began to feel that I was being called to help release that potential into the world, one patient at a time.

But something else happened during my training that influenced me to go into pediatric neurosurgery. I met more pediatric neurosurgeons—one in particular named Tim George. Because of a research project on brain imaging I had worked on with Tim at Duke, I went to a national meeting of pediatric neurosurgeons during my residency in order to present the work at the main session of the meeting. After a single day of hearing others speak at the microphone and meeting leaders and others who would one day become my mentors and then my peers, my wife, Melissa, a medical student at the time who had accompanied me to the meeting (her first too), turned to me and said, "You are among your people here." Literally, that is what she said, as if I were in a group of tourists in Wales and had just found out that I was Welsh.

It turns out we're a relatively small group. There are only around 250 or so of us across North America. Twenty percent of us are women, a higher number than for any other neurosurgical subspecialty. That number continues to grow, and we are clearly better off for it. Not surprisingly, we tend to the eccentric as well. At our national meetings when one of us begins to drone on and on at the lectern, there is a ceremonial gong that is enthusiastically banged, signaling *Enough!* I believe that we get along so well because we've lived the experience of taking care of kids who get well and kids who don't. Parents who are grateful to you or never want to see you again. Hours spent in the OR negotiating with a higher power for the bleeding to stop, the tumor to finally peel out, or the brain swelling to go down. *I'll do whatever you ask, God, please. Just help me get this thing out.*

Becoming a board-certified pediatric neurosurgeon requires an extra year after residency called a fellowship, and I decided to spend that year with a remarkable group led by a man named Jerry Oakes at the University of Alabama at Birmingham. He had been on faculty at Duke years before my time there and was highly regarded. Thankfully, there was much less conflict and more sleep in that year, despite the twelve-hour days. The hours spent in the operating room taught me many things, none more important as a surgeon than how the nervous system changes over time in its three-dimensional structure. The brain and surrounding structures of a premature infant are vastly different from those of an eighteen-year-old, and I came to understand the importance of time itself as the fourth dimension of anatomy, the sizes of structures, and the key relationships between them and the fragility of all of it growing, evolving, as a child ages. This would come to be a fundamental tenet of my teaching to the residents and medical students, and also a testament to the wondrous nature of the human nervous system.

Then you are done, eleven years after you graduated from college. Most wizened neurosurgeons would tell you that this time is when the real learning begins. When you are in charge, after you've finished your residency and become the attending, no one else scrubs in after you or walks in the hospital room or clinic room behind you. You are the one your patients and their parents trust; they see you as the way out of the nightmare that put them in front of you. I've been a pediatric neurosurgeon for nearly two decades now. I spent ten years in Birmingham and will soon complete ten years here at Vanderbilt. In the course of my career, I have done thousands of operations. Fetal operations are the most wondrous; trauma, when successful, the most gratifying. Tumors and vascular malformations are the hardest. Hydrocephalus the most routine, yet maddening when the smallest divergence from that routine brings about failure. I have made mistakes, have regrets, and also have some of the most wonderful memories that one could imagine. I have told families right before emergency surgery that I had to leave—*this is not a sit-down conversation,* I told one young couple after a ruptured brain aneurysm threatened their infant daughter's life—I just couldn't talk any longer, because I had to get into the OR to start saving their child. I've been yelled at, occasionally threatened when I couldn't stop the inevitable, and each time tried to understand how hard it was for the parents. I've cried with the parents from relief and sometimes from sadness. I've cried in the locker room when no one else was there and the tears welled up from a place I thought I had under control.

Years ago, I was asked to be involved in a case of recently born conjoined twins connected in the back of the heads who were very premature, so small and fragile. One was starting to get extremely ill from necrotic bowel—the intestines had started to die off, which can happen in extreme prematurity—and the blood toxins were threatening the other infant. We decided to try an emergency separation. Minimal films, dying children, no time for the weeks of preparation a case like this would normally take. It was a Hail Mary if ever there was one. Through the skin exposure and the craniotomy and then the dural opening, we'd lost less than a thimbleful of blood. All was going well, the vital signs were actually improving under anesthesia. But then, after three hours of surgery, as we worked deeper and deeper to separate the brains by coagulating the hundreds of tiny blood vessels connecting the two children, there was a little more bleeding. And then from down deep in the two connected brains there was a *lot* of bleeding; so much and we couldn't pack it off. The anesthesiologists were pushing blood into the twins' IV, and then all of a sudden I was cutting the joined skull with scissors, all hope of delicacy abandoned, trying to get them separated so that my partner and I could each take one and stop the bleeding.

And then the bleeding stopped.

It stopped because *all bleeding stops.* They had both died, and I remember that I couldn't see to sew and tears were falling onto the twin in front of me. I was sewing them up so that the parents could at least hold their babies one time, separated. We should have sacrificed the one for the other but we went for both and they were both gone and I still remember standing there unable to see.

For many years, I've kept an imaginary place just outside my vision, a plain field with very green grass. It came about out of necessity to give me a place to put these memories. When I would encounter something beyond comprehension, something that would cause me to question my faith or fill me with profound sorrow, I would sit quietly and think of that green field just outside my perspective. I would picture myself walking along the row of small mounds until I would find a new place, untouched. I would remove the sod and dig a hole in the ground and put the memory of that child whose story ended in sadness in a box. Then I would bury the box in the hole in the field and replace the sod and tamp it down to a little mound. Each time, I would do that. Then I would leave that green and walk back into life.

Then, in the summer of 2017, I watched as a CT scan scrolled on my computer screen as I had done thousands of times over the prior twenty-five years followed by a conversation about how it was a tumor and that there were different types, both benign and malignant, and that this looked malignant and we'd need to get some more images and then do surgery. This time, though, instead of my saying those things, it was me *hearing* them. There was a tumor the size of a racquetball in the muscle of my pelvis and upper leg, right over the nerve that controls your leg (*How many times have I exposed that very nerve?*), and it looked malignant, so I had a radical resection to take it out, and it did come out, along with some muscle necessary for walking around. Later I remember looking at it under the microscope with the pathologist so he could prove to me that it was benign, a one-out-of-a-*million* chance—the books actually said that. It was so odd to be looking at a part of yourself that had grown out of control. After the first surgery, there was a second to try to close the defect and then a third followed by strict bed rest. For ten weeks.

When you are on forced bed rest after having worked at warp speed for as long as you can remember, and you're feeling a little sorry for yourself, suddenly you realize, *Hey, it was benign, dumbass,* and it was not in the brain or spinal cord or chest or gut but in the muscle of the upper leg and that you will walk again one day, with therapy, and you begin to feel like you made it through an existential threat and that makes you think back through your life a little. And I remembered John Stone's note to me in the front of his book so many years before—"To Jay, at the beginning . . ."—and as I thumbed through that book while on bed rest, I thought about how I had gone to medical school to learn how to better understand life itself. And I thought of all the paths I had been privileged to cross since then, all the lessons I had learned.

It is not a surprise that we are all fragile. None more so than the littlest among us. The dark and unknown that we all face make us more so. But life wants to live, and I have learned that we are also extraordinarily resilient. None more so than the littlest among us. A child comes to us with a particular problem that requires intervention on the most sacred part of their being, the brain or spinal cord, those parts that make us essentially human. I most often feel that operating on them has had the effect of making me more essentially human, that as much as I have healed, I have been healed.

Now it is time to tell the stories of these remarkable children and our journeys together.

All That Moves Us

The Reminder

Throughout the spring of 2020, our hospital, like many others, was consumed with preparation for COVID-19. As colleagues on the West Coast affected by the earliest North American wave recounted their initial experiences via group call, social media, or text thread (*You can use an N95 respirator all day if you have to. You MUST double mask. Hoard your asthma inhalers. We've already gone down four nurses in the post-op recovery room who were exposed and are home in quarantine.*), the overall sense became bleak. Instead of performing surgery, I was tasked with sifting through rapidly incoming data (some valid, some not) as part of a perioperative committee that stood up to prepare for the anticipated surge of patients. Service teams were quickly boiled down to the most essential; operative procedures were canceled unless deemed urgent; all non-clinical personnel were sent home.

Into this, a twelve-year-old presented comatose with a ruptured brain arteriovenous malformation (AVM). A few hours earlier, she and her family had been following the state and local stay-at-home order by gathering to watch a Harry Potter movie marathon when she began to complain of a severe headache. Within minutes she was unresponsive.

This is the most challenging aspect of pediatric neurosurgery, the constant sense of impending calamity that spills over into your life outside work. Over the years, you become so conditioned to emergencies that the random becomes the reliable.

One minute it's popcorn and Harry Potter with the family, and then suddenly your daughter has the worst headache of her life and seizes from a brain hemorrhage.

Or a child eating breakfast before school slumps down into their cereal, the parents believing it's a gag until the terrible realization dawns that it's not.

Brakes on a bike that fail and into traffic your thirteen-year-old goes.

A father who turns his head while driving just to make sure his two-year-old's car-seat harness is on correctly, then runs off the road into a tree. Two days later he and his wife, still in neck braces and wheelchairs from the accident, have to make the decision to take their child, never to recover, off the ventilator.

These all roar at me in what must be normal moments for everyone else. A car seat was not just an inconvenient safety chore. It became as important to me as the moment the technicians would secure the Apollo astronauts into their safety harnesses before launch. Seeing my son jump helmetless onto a friend's skateboard spontaneously triggers memories of open depressed skull fractures rushed into the OR at 2:00 in the morning, someone's child's blood saturating my scrub pants all the way through until the material is pasted on my skin. Every moment in the car, every meal together, every time my children leave the house, if I let myself slide, I see the Jaws of Life, or a seizure, or a policeman knocking on my door.

At an emergency room near the twelve-year-old girl's home, a breathing tube had been inserted and mechanical ventilation was started, a lifesaving intervention to buy time. A CT scan had revealed a large blood clot inside the left frontal lobe of her brain pushing over to the right, and the hint of a small offending tangle of blood vessels, the AVM, just under the normally unperturbed surface. A doctor at the outside emergency room two and a half hours away had correctly made the diagnosis of a ruptured AVM and drilled a small hole through the skull to place a drain in the cerebral ventricles. This does two main things. It helps to reduce the pressure that can build up quickly inside the skull in situations like a brain hemorrhage, trauma, or a brain tumor, by physically draining the built-up CSF—cerebrospinal fluid—inside the brain. That drain also acts as a pressure monitor when connected to a bedside display. Having that number, the intracranial pressure, to follow then enables the nurses and doctors to infuse special intravenous medication that helps to lower that pressure and buy a little extra time for definitive care.

AVMs are among the most difficult operations we do. In normal circumstances, arteries are thick-walled and carry oxygenated blood under high pressure from the heart to the brain (and the rest of the body for that matter). That blood pressure then dissipates as the arteries continue to divide into smaller and more numerous arterioles and then finally until they turn into tiny capillaries. The capillary bed in most organs is made up of thousands of tiny vessels, each one the width of an individual red blood cell, and the oxygen within that cell is delivered through the capillary wall to the organ in need. That loss of oxygen is what causes the blood to lose its bright red color and turn darker, bluish. The deoxygenated bluish blood is under lower pressure on the other side of the capillary bed and begins to drain into larger and larger thin-walled veins that channel the blood back to the lungs for more oxygen and then to the heart for the pressure of the beating heart to propel the blood back along its way.

An AVM basically short-circuits that pathway. Typically present in a much smaller form since birth, these grow over time and can come to cause seizures, headaches, or even rupture acutely, like in this young girl. Instead of the normal pattern of flow from artery to vein through the capillary bed that dissipates the pressure evenly, those larger, high-pressure, thick-walled vessels containing oxygenated bright red blood drain directly into thin-walled veins that are not designed to handle the higher pressure coming from the heart. Over time, those thin-walled veins begin to collapse and coil around one another, the red blood jetting directly into the veins, arterializing the veins—making them red, angry, abnormal. Under the high magnification of the operating microscope, you can see the red and blue blood mixing and swirling through the vessels as the AVM pulses menacingly with each heartbeat.

When the outside physician called me before putting in the drain, it was just past midnight. The procedure and subsequent transfer took a few hours, and she arrived around 6:00 A.M. We brought her to the operating room soon afterward, first anesthesia and then the OR nurses converging on her quickly.

It's at this point, as we were set to proceed, that I had a way-too-quick talk with her mother about the possibilities. Often when patients arrive via emergency transport, they are given aliases just to quickly move through the electronic medical record and hospital system. This is when I learned from her mother that our patient's name was Sophia. I then had to tell her that Sophia could die or be permanently disabled from the initial AVM rupture, or she could die or be permanently disabled by the surgery to take it out. To be clear, permanently disabled means unable to move one side of her body, or mute, or alive on a machine, never to awaken. As I steel myself for conversations like these, while also focusing on the operative task at hand, I now find that I try to actively decouple the part of me who is a parent of children from the part of me who must operate on this very sick child. I imagine myself pressing on something like a clutch in my head in order to leave the parent part of my psyche spinning and disengaged from the surgeon. If I did not do this, then the concept of what this woman and all the parents over the years are going through at this very moment would become nearly overwhelming to consider. The truth is that I see it as a kind of weakness in these moments, one that a neurosurgeon should be able to keep under control. Letting my thoughts go, letting any control up, could undo me as I think back to first bike rides and soccer games and settling arguments and all the things that make up parenting of my own children.

I can fathom how hard this must be, and our whole team desperately wants to save your child, I promise. I want to tell you that everything is going to be all right and take away this pain you are feeling. But I need to decouple and to get down to the task at hand. Our best OR team is back there, and they've all been diverted to other things during this new COVID-19 era too, but now they are ready to get to work in the operating room. But in order to do that, we will all need to pull ourselves back just enough. Just enough to sterilize the operative field and drape one side of her head with towels and turn this person from your beloved daughter to a prepped-out rectangle, the person beneath otherwise covered in sterile drapes, so that all we will soon see is a window into the problem that we believe deeply we know how to solve.

The brain was tight with pressure from the underlying blood clot. It was tempting to remove the clot and reduce the pressure right off the bat. But the clot had stopped the bleeding by plugging up the hole in the ruptured blood vessel. Disrupting it off the ruptured vessel could restart the blood loss, and I did not want to risk that. Quickly, we found the offending artery feeding the AVM and exposed a few millimeters of it with micro-forceps. My resident, who was right beside me, carefully placed a tiny vascular clip across the artery. The moment she did, we saw a nearby engorged and pulsing draining vein turn from an angry swirling purple to a calm blue, signaling normalization of flow. One more tiny vascular clip placed across the vein directly exiting the AVM, and with a few cuts of the microscissors the AVM was out. We then carefully removed the blood clot from the deepest part of her brain, gently irrigating around it and letting it come to us, waiting near the surface with a tiny sucker to vacuum it out. Within a few seconds, the brain relaxed, the blood clot no longer exerting pressure from inside, and it was time to go.

As we worked to close up, I noticed an energy in the OR among our entire team that extended out beyond the room's doors and into the hallway. Colleagues checked in on us. Faces that normally would pass by appeared in the door window. I imagined all of it pent up from weeks of watching the world overcome by the relentless advance of this pandemic. Where we all were, there in that very moment of operating, was a reminder of our lives before, giving us clarity and purpose and a respite from the helplessness all of us felt as we watched our world change all around us. *We have healed in this OR before, and we will be able to heal again.*

I watched as Sophia recovered in the ensuing weeks after her surgery, awakening from her comatose state a few days later, then improving on a near-hourly basis: saying her family's names, reaching out for objects, interacting more and more with her environment. Soon she was transferred to a nearby rehabilitation hospital to focus on getting back to her feet. The brain pathways that she had worked out years ago when she learned to walk were still there; she just had to find them again. A few days later, instead of heading for my car at the end of a day in clinic, I walked across the street to the rehabilitation hospital and went for a visit.

By this point, the pandemic had settled in. New COVID-19 visitation restrictions kept her from having any visitors other than her parents, so they had been taking turns staying with her. I walked up to her open door and peered in before knocking on the frame to announce my presence. There she sat, not long ago on the verge of death, playing a game of cards with her mother. *A game of cards!* I thought back to my talk with her mom right before surgery. It was astounding. Even after years of doing this work that we were trained to do, of bringing children back from the edge, I am still washed over with wonder in these moments. Not only was she interactive and talking, but she was thriving. They both looked up at me from their cards and smiled. Her physical therapist came in soon after me, and I watched as she stood up from the edge of the bed to try her hand at walking again, still a challenge even with all the other improvements that had been going on. Her mom left her side, encouraging her as she did it, and came over to stand next to me. She watched as her mom easily walked across the room, then glanced back down, a look of determination coming across her face as she focused. I saw in her the resolution to be healed, to do her part in her recovery no matter how much it took out of her. I realized then, after enough weeks of this new pandemic life, how much I needed to witness her healing and her own willpower to do so. I thought how all of us in medicine needed to see this one child willing herself forward.

Slowly, steadily, Sophia put one foot out, her mother and I side by side at the door watching her. She gradually increased pressure on it as she got her balance. She dropped the therapist's steadying hand, deliberately, as if to say, *I can do this.* Next, just a little faster, came the other foot. Then the next step and the next until she was walking. Her mother reflexively squeezed my arm. It was as if we could see the neurons themselves waking up in front of us. Then, unexpectedly, Sophia walked right past us both out into the hall. With each step forward, bringing us all back to life.

———•◦•———

2

Stitches

I NEVER REMOVE STITCHES myself. It takes time. The kids are squirmy. It hurts them. Sometimes they yell, even cry. They never, ever like it. In fact, they fear it the way they fear shots. It's the most common question I get from the kids before surgery: "Will the stitches hurt?" So, I just don't do it. I am a brain surgeon. I've got brain surgeon stuff to do. I have someone else from my clinic come in and remove them at the two-week post-op check. Then, if I am in clinic or nearby, I can pop my head in the room and check on things once everything and everybody has calmed down.

Well into my second decade of practice, eight-year-old Dalayla presented with a severe headache, complete loss of vision, and a grapefruit-sized tumor on the left side of her brain, taking up nearly half of that side of her head and pushing the normal brain down and over to the opposite side. As brain tumors go, it was large and it was clearly causing a great deal of pressure on the surrounding tissue; her acute blindness was a symptom of that. I decided to take the tumor out in an urgent five-hour operation soon after she arrived. After clipping just enough of her black, beautifully braided hair to be able to sterilize the skin, we made a long S-shaped incision to expose the underlying bright white skull. Then we used a tiny drill to make small holes in the skull and connect them one by one to carefully remove a square window of bone overlying the tumor. The dura underneath was bulging out from the underlying pressure, and when we opened it with a tiny pair of scissors, the tumor and surrounding brain immediately began to swell outside the opening, pushing out into the empty space. We quickly began to gut the inner part of the tumor, creating a cavity on the inside so that we could carefully dissect the outside edges away from the surrounding brain. *Stay in the middle.* I always hear the voice of Jerry Oakes, a past surgical mentor, at this exact point. As the dissection plane between the tumor and the normal brain was developed, we placed tiny two-millimeter-thick cotton patties to help stanch the slow but steady venous ooze from the tumor. These cotton patties are absolute godsends for neurosurgeons, as we use them one by one to delineate normal from abnormal. We use so many of them during a single surgery, in fact, that there are tiny long blue strings that drape up and just over the edge of the craniotomy, so that we can see them and don't leave one in inadvertently. The nurses and scrub techs meticulously count them at the end just to make sure. We do *not* want to leave something inside the head that we do not mean to. We brought in the operating microscope to help see as we separated the edges of the tumor from the normal surrounding brain. As we worked, I could see tiny thrombosed blood vessels and what looked like dead tumor in the core, indicating that the tumor was growing so fast it was outgrowing its own internal blood supply—a concerning sign of malignancy.

We couldn't dwell on this, though. We were millimeters away from the motor strip. Time passed as the resident and I worked. As more and more tumor came out, the bleeding began to slow down, and the brain around the tumor began to relax. Once we had the last portion out, the brain had filled in at least half of the cavity already. *Happy,* I thought, *to have the invader out.* Then I remembered that we too were invaders, and we made our own way out, careful to repair each layer—dura, bone, skin—with each step.

As Dalayla woke up from anesthesia in the operating room, the scrub nurses carefully removed the instruments and tools from around her in order to clean and ready them for another day. She flickered her eyes open as the sedation gradually wore off. She reached up to shield her eyes from the bright lights of the OR. *A good sign.* We held our breath. Someone held up two fingers in front of her. She counted them both. *But everyone guesses two, I thought.* I held up first a pen. "Pen," she said. Then object after object. "Phone, thumb, watch," she said, naming them as I pulled all sorts of things out to show her. The anesthesiologist patted me on the shoulder and moved to inject just enough sedation for transport to the ICU. "I think we've seen enough, Jay," she said, smiling. "Let's get her upstairs. What do you think?" I nodded. We were convinced. I was convinced. She could see.

The scrub nurse looked up from her work counting the instruments before sending the trays out of the room.

"Hallelujah."

I went out to find her mother, Leslie, in the waiting room. She saw me the moment I came through the door, stepping away from her large family, anxious, her eyes searching my face for any sign of good news. I told her that the tumor was out, that Dalayla had woken up neurologically intact, and that she could see. I held up my pen and thumb and watch as proof, telling her how she had named them and how the anesthesiologist had to finally call me off. Her mother reached out to touch the pen. She stared at it for a moment, her hand hanging there between us, then she hugged me. After a few seconds, she turned to hug her family. They formed a circle and offered prayers for the news, and I joined them for a moment, hesitant to invade their sacred space with the knowledge I had in my brain. I remember Leslie standing across from me with her head bowed, a loving and calm force for her child, steeling herself to take on this next challenge in their life together.

In my mind, as we stood there in prayer, all I could see were those tiny thrombosed blood vessels in the middle of the tumor, the necrotic part in the center. There I stood, in the circle, hold-ing hands with the family, eyes closed. I was not giving thanks for her recovered vision but asking for a miracle. A miracle that I was wrong and that the tumor was benign, not malignant. But I knew I was not. Nothing would change the fact that the frozen section of tumor sent to pathology from the OR was thought to be a glio-blastoma multiforme, a GBM—a grade 4 out of 4 tumor, highly malignant and never fully curable. The average life expectancy for a child with that tumor type is one to two years, and its growth tends to be relentless once it recurs. The final pathologic diagnosis would not be back for a few days, and for the moment I had to separate the wake-up from surgery from my eventual duty to tell parents the final pathologic diagnosis. But that moment was coming.

By the second day after surgery, Dalayla was sitting up in bed, cracking jokes with her family. The next day, she had the nurses and our rounding team laughing at nearly her every word. She held on to a ukulele and threatened to play it unless we would do some task of her choosing, like change her lunch order to all ice cream or bring her comic books to read. Her resilience and remarkable spirit in the aftermath of such a profound surgery inspired all of us in our work.

"How you doing, Dr. Jay?" she would ask me as I walked by to check on her at the end of a long day. "You look tired. You need to get more sleep!" she would say, and then I would pretend to conk out in the middle of our conversation. Laughter all around.

The evening before discharge, I walked in to talk to Leslie about the final results from pathology and pulled a chair over to sit away from Dalayla, who at that point had headphones on, listening to music. I do wonder what Dalayla saw while she sat there in bed lis-tening to the music. Me leaning forward in the chair, talking to her mother, a concerned look on my face. Her mother putting her own face in her hands and crying. Me clumsily offering a paper towel in lieu of a tissue, the nearby box on the sink edge empty. Us sitting quietly for a while afterward, then me standing up. With a hand on her mother's shoulder and a few more words, I was gone. Their world forever changed.

After discharge, Dalayla and her energy were missed. I knew that she had returned for her sutures to be removed because I saw Leslie in the hall of our clinic. I was careful to wait until the nurses had finished taking her stitches out before I walked in to inquire about her ukulele-playing skills. Leslie was standing by her side, smiling. We chatted for a bit, and I gave further instructions about wound care, probably too much as I always did. We set a follow-up for the future, but gradually, over the next year, her care shifted away from us and to the oncology outpatient team.

As predicted, but a little faster than expected, the tumor came back. This time at the surface of the brain and involving the dura (which is typically immune from GBM) and even the bone (nearly unheard of) and behaving even more aggressively than ever expected. When I saw them both, there was no ukulele in sight. We made plans for another tumor resection. Neither had any questions, trusting me that what I would do would be fine. After the surgery consent form had been signed, her mother and I spontaneously embraced. I told her how sorry I was that the tumor had come back.

Later that week, we took the recurrence out, including the dura and enough of the involved bone that we needed to place some mesh and bone paste to fill the half-dollar-sized hole so she wouldn't have an obvious defect under her bald scalp. This time around, after surgery, Dalayla was quieter. A year of living each day with a brain tumor, with the chemotherapy and radiation along the way, had changed her. This time, there was no prayer circle. Only Mom, present, strong, constant, at her side.

Within three weeks, she returned with an infection of the graft material. Her immune system was compromised, making her far more susceptible to infection, yes, but the surgeon who chooses to blame a complication on the patient's condition is fooling him-

or herself entirely. Infection can come from several sources, some surgeon-controlled, like a contamination at the time of surgery or a lapse in diligence in wound closure, and some not surgeon-controlled, such as a urine or blood infection. Often, it's never exactly known. Regardless, most of us feel it as our own.

Far worse than that, however, she had tumor recurrence all over her brain. From adjacent to the area of surgery, to the crevices of the multiple temporal lobe folds on the opposite side, to all along its base where it rested on the skull. The white of the tumor on the MRI appeared like a disfigured hand wrapping its fingers around the gray of the brain, squeezing her life away ever so slightly more with each passing day. There was no way to control its relentless growth. No more surgery, chemotherapy, or even radiation therapy would make a difference. There was no way to prolong her life in a meaningful way. It was time to reset our priorities, an all too familiar place for those of us who deal with pediatric brain tumors. Treatment turned to palliation. Conversations with her mother turned from curing her disease to controlling her pain and allowing her to live the remainder of her days with as little discomfort as possible.

We took her to the operating room one last time and removed the small piece of mesh and bone paste, then gently washed out the area where the infection was. It was not as severe as I had thought, my initial impression likely worsened by my guilt at the possibility that I had added yet more to this child's burden, and two weeks of oral antibiotics cleared up any sign of infection. At the two-week mark, when we usually see children back in clinic for the dreaded suture removal, she had been readmitted to the oncology service to try to better control the pain from the tumor spreading down along her spinal cord. We saw her that day, and the wound was healing well. My team made plans to remove her sutures and save her an extra clinic visit. As we finished up rounds, I thought about how it was unlikely that I would ever see Dalayla or her mother again after this visit. Soon she would be leaving for a trip to Disney World, funded by the Make-A-Wish Foundation and expedited due to her terminal condition. As she lay quietly in bed, her eyes closed and her face nearly still as she spoke, we talked a little about why Wonder Woman wasn't a Disney character (yet), her planned princess breakfast, perhaps a ride or two if she felt like it.

I decided right then to remove her stitches myself. In fact, I desperately wanted no one else to do it. It was my job to do, mine alone. A way for me to say goodbye to her more familiar than saying the words out loud.

She was tired—sleepy from the morphine given to help her pain. When I came back in, her mother helped her roll away from me so I could get to the wound. I carefully clipped each stitch, the movements as slight as my nearly twenty years as a micro-neurosurgeon could afford. With a series of the tiniest tugs, each one was out. She did not squirm or cry. Her mother sat next to her holding her hand. On occasion, while I was concentrating, Leslie would turn her own face away to quietly cry in the direction of the TV so Dalayla would think she had been distracted by something playing above them.

When I was done, I carefully gathered up the scissors, the forceps, and each of the removed sutures and bundled them up in gauze to take with me out of the room. Leslie and I caught each other's gaze and she mouthed "Thank you" to me. I looked at her for a moment, said my goodbyes, wished Dalayla a wonderful trip to Disney World, and walked out.

As I left the ward, I quickly entered the nearest empty conference room, shut the door, and sat down, my head in my hands. I am aware that I have never completely known this deep aching pain of losing a child and beg desperately each night that I never have to. But in my time as a surgeon, I have sat next to it, held its hand, and turned my head away to cry over and over and over.

3

———•+•———

The Brain and All That Moves Us

OME ON, WHAT'S it really like? Is it like jelly? Or a melon? What about the color? What color is it?"

"Yogurt," I say. "Crème-colored vanilla yogurt." Then I smile and continue for effect. "The really thick stuff where the spoon stands up in it."

"Eeewwwwww . . . ," the kids say and run away laughing as the adults roll their eyes, everyone at once repelled at and fixated on the idea that the brain is like thick vanilla yogurt and anybody would even consider putting a spoon in it.

When people find out that my workplace is the human brain, they all want to know what it looks like; they want to know its color and its consistency. *No, I have not touched it without gloves on. Really?* Kids at work, friends of my own kids who gather up the nerve to ask, even adults at our middle school parent social night. Everyone, it would appear, except my wife.

"What's the big deal?" my wife, Melissa, the now-endocrinologist, said when she rotated through neurosurgery as a medical student at Duke. I was on a mandatory neurology rotation for the month, so the faculty and other residents hammed it up in my absence. They had her helping to drill burr holes for removing chronic subdural hematomas (long-standing blood clots most common in the elderly and responsible for confusion and seizures, among other symptoms) and scrubbing in to OR cases of all sorts. All while having her make it home by 6:00 P.M. It was like a big gaslight-by-proxy pointed directly at me.

"Neurosurgery is not that hard, sweetie," she would tell me upon my return. "You guys just make it out to be that way to keep it all mysterious."

Well, damn it, the brain is mysterious (stomping feet)! Melissa's tongue-in-cheek comment aside, there is so much yet to be fully divined about its secrets. This organ of mostly protein and fat somehow allows us to interact with the world around us and makes us who we are. What is known of the brain and nervous system? Let's set the stage for answering that by "bringing in the scope"—a term we use when we rotate the operating microscope over the surgical field so that we can begin to unfold the secrets hidden along and under the brain's surface. Take a moment here to peer into the brain's mysteries through the eyes of a neurosurgeon.

Consider yourself now standing at the head of the table, positioned just over the patient's exposed brain. Long blue sterile drapes cover all but the area of focus. The hiss of the ventilator and rhythmic tones of the heart monitor are the only sounds in the background. The room is otherwise silent, the lights now turned down in preparation for the microscope to be brought into place. The overlying skull has been carefully removed. The dura, the leathery covering of the brain, has been opened and flapped back out of the way. The OR team has moved the heavy base of the operating microscope into place next to the patient; the actual microscope itself hangs up and over the patient on a series of levers like cranes swinging into a construction zone. It is wrapped in a sterile drape and perfectly balanced so that the tiniest movement is all it takes to adjust its viewing angle. Triggers on the handles off to its sides allow you to adjust its position, focus in and out, and turn the brightness up and down. This microscope will be your window into another reality. In a moment, time will dilate as your focus narrows, your breath-

ing slows, and distractions fall into the distance. You peer forward
into the eyepieces, and your gaze is directed straight down onto the
surface of the brain, to a scene the likes of which only few have
encountered, initially as alien as the moonscape must have been
to its early visitors. Except instead of desolate grayness all around,
the brain's surface is bursting with color and light, with dimension
and depth. It takes a moment for your eyes to adjust to the sudden brightness. The surface is smooth and indeed crème-colored,
with just the faintest tint of yellow. It glistens from the microscope's
reflected light and is covered in a fine network of blood vessels and a
thin veil of translucent tissue called the arachnoid layer that reminds
you of plastic wrap. There are crevices called sulci, in between them
the gyri, and all following standard patterns along the surface. In
and around them you can predict the position of the motor strip—
the area that controls movement (hint: super important)—as well as
sensation (ditto), vision (ditto), speech (very ditto), and the whole
universe of things that the brain does.

When a neurosurgeon has to go through part of the brain to find
a tumor, or blood vessel malformation, or whatever we're going
after, we use a pair of delicate bayoneted forceps, called a bipolar
for the electrical current that passes through its tips when triggered,
in order to coagulate a few millimeters of the brain's surface and
also the tiny blood vessels along with it. Then, with a bayoneted pair
of microscissors, we cut the tiny blood vessel and the coagulated
surface of the brain, just enough to carefully get your dissector into
the opening as well as a little metal suction tube in your other hand.
The dissector comes in different microscopic shapes and sizes and
the one used is likely determined as much by the place that you
trained to become a neurosurgeon as by anything else. The suction
in the other hand has a tiny slit where it rests in your upturned palm
that you can cover with your thumb to regulate the amount of aspi-
ration power. These four instruments—the bipolar, the suction, the
microscissors, and the dissector—are the most common tools used

by a neurosurgeon when working in the brain or spinal cord itself. If ever there was a starter kit for neurosurgeons, perhaps to be rolled up in a little leather kit for the inside jacket pocket, it would consist of these four.

Once we pass through the slightly firmer brain surface and gradually make our way down to the lesion, we move carefully through the surrounding gray matter, where most of the cell bodies of the neurons reside, then into the white matter where the millions of the brain's connecting tendrils, the axons, exist. We use the suction and dissector here in a way that reminds me of sculpting, the way the finest little swipes help to form the tract as we advance deeper and deeper to then carefully sculpt out the tumor or AVM or lesion.

The brain and nervous system as I have come to see it have a dual nature. There is the anatomy around which we as neurosurgeons navigate in the operating room (or in our dreams in the nights and days before challenging cases) and how that surface anatomy relates to the internal neuroanatomy of the brain—the "wiring" or connectivity of the neurons and axons that defines who we are and how we move through this world. Taken together, these are what I consider the literal brain.

Then there is that metaphorical version—some would label this the mind—the spiritual or mystical brain that has inspired humankind since the realization of its existence. (This may or may not include the ancient Egyptians, who were mixed on the topic. It is known that they removed the intracranial contents—that is, the brain—through the nose after death, figuring that it was not an important structure, doing so as they carefully saved every other organ for burial. Yet their understanding of severe cranial and spinal cord injury is well documented in the Edwin Smith Papyrus as an "ailment not to be treated." Truly an astounding document to read through a modern lens.)

The brain is the seat of the soul, where self-awareness originates. It's how we define our self versus our not-self. It is why we have the ceiling of the Sistine Chapel, the poetry of Maya Angelou, or the beauty that surrounds us in the impressionism exhibits displayed in the Art Institute of Chicago. Of course, it is also how we have *Mein Kampf,* the Tulsa Race Massacre of 1921, and the Bataan Death March. Because of the complex interactions occurring in the brain, we grow to create and destroy, attack or defend, love and hate. It remains the most powerful (and mysterious!) structure in known existence.

Cerebrum

The brain has two main sides—the two hemispheres—divided up into lobes that are responsible for thought, speech, sensation, movement, vision, memory, and all the things that make us sentient. Below the surface of the brain are critical nuclei, microscopic aggregations of cells that coordinate movement, serve as a relay station for the senses as they travel up from the body, and maintain the fight-or-flight reflex and other critical "housekeeping" functions of the brain—breathing, heartbeat, temperature control, and more. All of these are interconnected with millions of neurons and supplied by a dense tree of blood vessels, critical for oxygen delivery, and hence survival of the brain cells, most of which are called neurons.

Years ago, I remember a remarkable teenager, Hannah, who began to have the slightest tremor of her right hand. She covered it up initially, as we are all wont to do, not wanting her friends to see her hand shaking or her parents to worry. But it began to awaken her at night. Soon the trembling was obvious even underneath the jacket or sweater she would wrap around it. Hannah's parents—her mom is a wellness coach and personal trainer—noticed quickly that something was wrong and began the search for why. The MRI ultimately ordered by their family doctor revealed a walnut-sized tumor in the basal ganglia—the deep nuclei of the brain responsible for coordinating movement—on the left side of her brain, and a large cyst

associated with the tumor pressing on all of the surrounding structures. Suddenly her high school sports were stopped, her soon-to-
be-gained driver's license was forgotten, and her college search was
set aside. Her entire life was put on hold until a plan could be made.

I met her and her parents, and we discussed the risks of surgery. The tumor was down next to several important blood vessels
in the base of the brain, and that large cyst was compressing the
all-important basal ganglia. After an intense conversation, Hannah
looked up and told me that she trusted me and wanted to return to
school as soon as possible. She had her life to get back to, after all.
Then she hugged her parents and the decision was made.

I remember how, under the microscope, the tumor was surrounded by the tiny blood vessels passing up into the normal
brain, like a beaded curtain draped over the lesion. We opened and
removed the cyst under the operating microscope. Then we began
to remove the tumor from the encircling vessels. Several of the tiny
vessels passed into the edge of the tumor just underneath the surface and traveled out the other end, to the normal brain. We took
our time and carefully dissected the vessels away from the tumor
and ensured each vessel was clear of tumor. One, slightly deeper
than the others, began to bleed as we attempted to separate it from
the tumor. The vessel was encased, and if the tumor was going to
come out, it would have to be coagulated and cut. So that's what we
did. It was the smallest of all of them and all the rest had been left
fully intact. Experience had told me that she had plenty of blood
supply preserved going to the surrounding important brain. When
we were done, I saw no residual tumor, and the brain was more
relaxed. After the dura was closed and the skull plate replaced, I
went out to speak with the parents, pleased with the day's events.
That would soon change.

I entered the consultation room outside the OR with a smile on
my face. I sat down, shaking their hands as I did. Just as I was telling them that the procedure went fine, I received a text message

that she wasn't waking up as expected. In fact, she wasn't moving one side. At all. I looked up from my phone, excused myself, and re-entered the OR. I watched as Hannah, instead of opening her eyes and following commands—what I expect for a wake up after surgery—barely moved her right side. Not only was the tremor gone, but all movement of that arm. Her leg was weaker than the other side as well. An emergency MRI showed a tiny stroke, literally a pinpoint on the screen—a sign that the very blood vessel we had to coagulate was likely a main branch supplying the basal ganglia, despite all the other vessels. There was no way to go back and reverse what had been done. Walking back out to update the family was difficult. There were no smiles as I sat down. After the news I told them that only time would tell the fullness of her injury and the ultimate degree of her recovery. I knew that this would take a great deal of time.

It took Hannah months to recover her movement on that side. In truth, it took her some time to regain the same level of cognition as before. There remains a permanent area of blindness in her vision due to involvement of a nearby visual tract, which relays information from the eye to the occipital lobe, where the interpretation of those signals resides. But now, years later, she has not only recovered; she has excelled. There are residual issues. She drives with a modified vehicle to a local college where she pushes herself to take the hardest classes. Her tremor remains gone, but she has permanent mild weakness of that hand, a high price to have paid for tumor removal. If you ask her, she is nonplussed. "This is my life," she says. "We are put here to make the best of things." Each challenge is just one more thing for her to push past, to overcome. She is a remarkable young woman. Her mother feels like she could not have had a better career in preparation to help their daughter recover, and she has been generous with information on Hannah's experience to help other patients that came after her.

Over the years, we've all developed a strong bond. Hannah was one of the first of my patients for me to see in follow up after I returned from my own muscle tumor resection a year or so after her own. I took from her the idea of naming my tumor after I was diagnosed. Hannah's was Li'l Devil, and in following an underworld motif, I had named mine Wormwood, after a C. S. Lewis character from *The Screwtape Letters* whose sole purpose was to bring about the fall of man. I proudly showed her the tennis ball—the size of my tumor—with the name Wormwood that I had written on it and stared at while I was on three months of bed rest before I was able to learn to walk again. She loved it. Of course, her parents still send me exercises.

Cerebellum

In terms of tumors and blood vessel malformations in the pediatric population, the back of the brain, called the cerebellum, is where pediatric neurosurgeons tend to do a good bit of our intracranial work. In addition to congenital malformations that can occur there that can require surgery, for a reason yet to be discerned, tumors and blood vessel malformations of the cerebellum are much more common in children. This lobe of the brain sits in the back of the head, also with two main hemispheres. The cerebellum's major role is in coordination as well, working in direct connection to the basal ganglia discussed above. The cerebellum is key in what it takes to learn to write, swing a golf club, hit a baseball, or spin pasta onto a fork. In the early days of neuroanatomy, it was the under-regarded smaller sibling of the cerebrum; neuroscientists are reported to have routinely discarded it when studying the brain. In addition to coordinating movement throughout the body, the cerebellum is believed to enable the coordination of speech and even of thought. As the frontal lobes have grown over the course of evolution from early mammal to simian to human, so have the lateral lobes of the cerebellum, likely taking on a greater role as we began to think and communicate on increasingly higher planes.

Because of where the cerebellum sits, in the back of the head, tumors that grow over either months or weeks can block the normal flow of cerebrospinal fluid through the brain, causing a syndrome called hydrocephalus in which brain pressure is elevated due to the inability of the fluid to escape. Hydrocephalus is the most common entity that we deal with as pediatric neurosurgeons. The development of the ventriculoperitoneal shunt—a tubular device that diverts the obstructed fluid through a tube under the skin into the abdomen—in the mid-1950s is responsible for saving tens of thousands of lives yearly of children or adults who would otherwise die. It is impossible to mention the field of neurosurgery without mentioning the role of the shunt both in saving children's lives and in the rise of pediatric neurosurgery as a field separate from adult neurosurgery. Indeed I can imagine that my national and international pediatric neurosurgery colleagues will be amazed that it took me this long to mention hydrocephalus at all.

But for lesions of the cerebellum the treatment is typically not placement of a shunt unless hydrocephalus remains after tumor or vascular lesion removal. Definitive treatment is resection when possible, and these presentations tend to be one of worsening headaches or vomiting for weeks or even months. Then brain imaging, urgent phone calls, and consultations with neurosurgeons happen, followed by resection.

In situations when there is an acute rupture of a vascular abnormality, like an AVM or cavernous malformation, the development of hydrocephalus is not gradual but rapid. Rapid and urgent and deadly if untreated.

Megan was an eight-year-old who woke up early one morning with a terrible headache. Within minutes she sat up to vomit, then fell over into her mother's arms and became unresponsive. After a frantic 911 call, an ambulance arrived to take her to our children's hospital emergently. En route, she began to seize and her heart rate became unstable. Ninety minutes after all of this began, Megan was wheeled into our trauma bay in the ED, where a large team had gathered in anticipation of her arrival.

She was close to death. Her rapid CT scan showed a large blood clot in her cerebellum causing hydrocephalus. We suspected a ruptured cavernous malformation, a vascular lesion similar to an AVM, but there was no time for an MRI or further imaging. Our senior neurosurgery resident placed a drain in her brain right there in the trauma bay to drain off the fluid and relieve the pressure that had built up. Minutes after she was done, Megan stirred. But still the clot was too large. We quickly decided to get her up to the operating room, turned her prone, shaved the back of her head, and proceeded to open the skin over the back of the head, remove the overlying bone, and take out the plum-sized blood clot that was pressing on her brain. The moment we took it out, her vital signs began to normalize.

After surgery, Megan opened her eyes in the ICU and tracked her mom walking around the bed. But she couldn't lift her arms without a pronounced tremor. Once recovered enough to be off the breathing machine, she didn't speak. It was like she could not coordinate the effort to do it. She couldn't sit up, her body shimmying from lack of control. We had saved her life, but this state was difficult for her and her mother and heartbreaking for us to see. *What had we brought her back into?* Fortunately, Megan was a child with the same immense potential for recovery that most children have. Also fortunately, Megan had her mother, who never left her side, who willed her through rehabilitation out of state, and who remains a force for adequate resources for children of all ages to have access to rehabilitation centers after brain injury.

I last saw Megan at a local triathlon. She was the symbolic first competitor, and I saw her with her number one race bib headed off for the swim. I realized quickly that she was symbolic in name only. Megan was there to win. I cheered with her mother when she crossed the finish line, and I stood amazed—*amazed!*—as Megan told my children, in her own words, of her ordeal. And then of my role in it. My daughter, Fair, looking back and forth from Megan, a girl her age, to me, for the first time saw the reality behind the stories that she occasionally heard at the dinner table as to why Dad had to leave. Megan, her mother, and I remain close as they send me photos of her continued milestones and I get to watch her grow into the young woman she was meant to be.

Brainstem

Just as the stem of a mushroom sits underneath the cap, the brainstem is the portion of the brain that sits underneath the cerebrum and in front of the cerebellum. Divided from top down into the midbrain, pons, and medulla, the brainstem has several critical nuclei of its own in addition to serving as a highway for the various motor and sensory tracts that pass to and from the spinal cord. These nuclei are responsible for much of what we deem is the role of the face, head, and neck, and are grouped as the cranial nerves, numbered I through XII.

It is important here to mention the deadliest of tumors in children, the DIPG—diffuse intrinsic pontine glioma—which occurs in this tightly packed space. These children present with eye and facial movement issues, often weakness from the motor tract involvement passing to the spinal cord. The imaging ultimately done in response to these symptoms reveals the death sentence of a DIPG. Surgery is impossible: The tumor is intimately interwoven into the dense and critical structures of the pons. Radiation and chemotherapy together impart just over a one-year survival at best. Burned into my memory from my residency days is the mother of a twelve-year-old girl about to be told that her daughter has been diagnosed with a DIPG. They were in the clinic of one of my attending pediatric neurosurgeons, Herb Fuchs. Herb is very much the same now as he was then, tall and skinny, with a tendency to tell the same story over and over, and loved by his patients. Once he had finished examining the girl, he subtly motioned for me to lead her out to sit with the nurses. As I did so, I noticed that she was a bit unsteady on her feet. I also remember looking back through the door as it was closing behind me to see Herb staring down at the ground. I know now he was gathering his nerve for what was to come. When I returned to the room minutes later, the mother had grabbed him by the lapels and was shaking him, sobbing that her daughter wanted to grow up to be a Supreme Court justice and how in God's name could he be telling her this. I remember him reaching out to gently embrace her until her heaves subsided. A moment later the woman stepped away to dab her eyes, regain control, and turn headlong into her fresh nightmare.

When I see Herb today, closing in on retirement, always asking me how the better Dr. Wellons is doing—meaning my wife—I remember that very moment. I remember her pain, his grace, and the brief aftermath that I witnessed. I find myself, even now, hoping to live up to his example of how we are to show compassion and even love in the midst of the great and nearly unbearable pain that we must at times unleash upon our patients.

Meninges and Skull

The brain is surrounded and protected by the dura mater—Latin for "tough mother"—that leathery material covering the surface of the brain. It must be opened sharply with a knife or scissors and reflected back in order to access the intracranial contents. The major traumatic hemorrhages are named based on the relationship to the dura. An epidural hematoma is outside the dura and below the bone. Its formation is usually due to a laceration to an artery that traverses the outside of the dura. Alternatively, the blood can be subdural and is usually associated with bleeding from a torn vein coming directly from the brain itself. Most of the time, the injury to the surrounding brain with a subdural hematoma tends to be much worse, the road to recovery substantially longer.

Just underneath the dura is the arachnoid membrane. This is that fine plastic wrap–like substance that covers the brain alluded to earlier. Within it is contained the cerebrospinal fluid once it has made its way outside the brain itself. The arachnoid has fine septations that are predictable so that small pockets of CSF, called cisterns, are opened on their way to exposing the various regions of the brain. The final membrane covering the brain surface is the pia. This is responsible for the glistening of the brain's surface. It runs up and down each and every crevice and is intimately adherent to the brain's surface. The role of the pia is less understood, but it is what was gently coagulated at the very beginning of our story earlier, and there, just over the cortical surface of the brain and the underlying tumor, we remain poised until our anatomy lesson is complete.

Protecting all of it is the skull. The skull is fascinating in that it is made up of multiple plates of bone allowing brain growth as a child. Then, as that growth slows, the bones come together over time, like tectonic plates, and seal up to form the skull. For kids under four, the skull is thinner, one layer, and tends to bend a little more than it breaks. Over four, and the bone begins to thicken, forming three layers: the denser bone on the surfaces and, sandwiched between, the trabecular bone, in which blood circulates within the skull. In order to get to the brain, we have to drill holes through the skull, then connect them with what is best described as a handheld band saw, in a very simplistic 1-2-3-4 square version of connect the dots. At the end of most brain operations we must replace the bone, so we secure the bone "flap" back to the skull with tiny little metal or plastic plates, the size of clipped fingernails. Over time, the bone knits itself back up again, never quite as strong as before, but just strong enough.

Spinal Cord

The brainstem narrows as it approaches the base of the skull, like an inverted pyramid, and exits through the hole at the base of the skull called the foramen magnum to become the spinal cord. The "cord" remains part of the central nervous system and contains the cell bodies and axons of over a million neurons running to and from all parts below the head.

The spinal cord, like the brain, is covered by the dura. Examining a cross section of the spinal cord at any level would show the axons running to the nerves innervating the muscles of the body to cause movement, as well as sensory fibers carrying pain, temperature, or position sense back to the brain. When a patient is in an accident that results in quadriplegia, it means that their arms, trunk, and legs are weak or paralyzed with limited to no sensation, depending on the severity of the injury, and the cervical spine is the level injured. For those with normal arm function, but none to very little in the legs or pelvis, the level of the lesion is more likely in the thoracic or lumbar spine, and that patient is referred to as having paraplegia. The difference in quality of life and need for long-term assistance between the two is tremendous.

Protecting all of it is the bony spine, known as the spinal column, a series of articulating bones held together by ligaments and muscles. Over time, these bony joints can wear down with osteoarthritis or be prone to herniation of the soft tissue disks between the vertebral bodies. Traumatic injury or loss of calcium causing osteoporosis can contribute to spine fracture, all of these possibly resulting in arm or leg pain or symptoms of spinal cord compression. It is rare for someone to have an injury causing quadriplegia or paraplegia without significant injury to the spinal column as well. One of the key roles of surgeons who operate on the spine, be it pediatrics or adults, in addition to removing compressive lesions like herniated disks or tumors involving the cord or column, is to understand how to effectively piece the spinal column back together in a way that can promote spinal cord healing if injured as well as ensure stability of the bony column.

For now, there remains no cure for spinal cord injury. While level of care immediately afterward and aggressive rehabilitation are important, severity of the initial injury remains the biggest predictor of recovery. Having to tell parents that their child is forever in a wheelchair or, worse, on a ventilator because of a high cervical spine injury—after the football tackle that went awry, or the sledding accident that took them into a tree, or the split-second decision to dive headfirst off a swing rope into a murky shallow pond—is a part of pediatric neurosurgery that I and every single one of my colleagues wish gone, solved, and cured forever. But sometimes, in particular emergency situations involving the spine, you have the chance to jump in and make a difference ultra-early.

Just like in the brain, tumors and AVMs can occur in and around the spinal cord. What is it like to have the chance to help someone walk again? When, without stepping in to do something, it would be gone forever? To be clear, I'm talking about hearing that particular ping on your phone you have for emergencies, looking down to see the images scrolling across on the screen, excusing yourself from dinner, and returning the call on the drive to the hospital.

This exact scenario occurred recently while visiting a friend's home for dinner for the first time in a year.

"Good evening, Dr. Wellons." The voice coming from my car speakers as I pull onto the street is from the fourth-year neurosurgery resident on call with me for the night. She and I had worked together a good bit, and I had come to see that she misses very little. I still like it when we are on call together.

"We've got a three-year-old girl who's been progressively weaker in the legs over the last two days," she said. "I'm outside her room and just examined her. She really can't move them much at all for me. Lots of crying with attempts at weight bearing. Parents are clearly worried."

She continues, "The MRI shows a large epidural blood clot along the five levels of the thoracic spine. The spinal cord is clearly compressed, but I don't see an obvious cause of the clot on the scan."

The blood has collected between the dura, the covering of the spinal cord, and the bony roof of the spinal canal. It is indenting the underlying spinal cord significantly. Swelling and a lack of blood flow of the cord can be seen on the emergent MRI that was just completed. This matches with the paralysis of the legs. It's rare for a three-year-old to have this without an explanation. I file away the fact that it may be a tumor or blood vessel abnormality, something to be mindful of in the OR.

"What do you think we should do?" I say now, two minutes away from the parking deck and fully committed for the night, thinking through how long this should take and if it will affect my ability to do my cases the next day.

"I think we need to decompress it," she says assuredly.

"When?" I ask, fully knowing the answer.

"Tonight," she says back quickly.

"Right answer," I say.

She continues, "It could be an odd spinal AVM, but we don't really have time for an angiogram. The faster we get the pressure off, the higher chance that she will walk again."

"I agree. No matter what it is, tumor, AVM, spontaneous clot, it is coming out," I say. "Let the OR know that I am driving in."

"I already did," she says, and I notice now that she is slightly out of breath. "I could hear you driving, so I took the stairs while we were talking and confirmed with the OR team that we were a go.

They are setting up now. Anesthesia is aware and going to get her. The parents will be waiting for you in the waiting room."

As I said, she misses very little.

I spoke with the mother and father soon afterward. We stood at the doors to the OR. Their child was the only emergency operation of the night for any surgical service at this point, so things were moving quickly, tremendously beneficial to her and her chance to walk again.

Right then I needed to let them know how critical surgery was. As all of us are wont to do, the parents began to tell me the story of how they told the first doctor two days ago that something was wrong but because there was no real weakness, they were sent home. Then at the emergency department at an outside hospital they said it again . . . and as I have had to do in the past in these situations, when the families want to include every detail in case it could help in some way, I had to politely step in and stop them.

"Mom and Dad," I said, "I want to hear this, I really do, but I need to get going."

They stopped talking and looked at me silently. I had to make sure they were aware that I was not a complete ass, but that I had to get started if their daughter was going to have a chance to walk again.

Non-acute neurological decline in a young child can be difficult to detect until things progress to the obvious. I've seen kids come in nearly fully blind who in retrospect had been sitting closer and closer to the TV until Mom comes in to see them with their face one inch away from the screen. Same thing for arm weakness in an infant, as the other arm works as a buddy to help lift bottles and blocks. With leg movement in particular, it's hard in the early stages of weakness. Who hasn't seen a crying toddler not want to put pressure on their legs and just collapse during a fit. Once the seriousness of things is realized, most parents become distraught that they missed something. Some become angry at their pediatrician or primary care doctor for "missing it." My approach has always been to assuage any of that. All of us don't want things to be the worst possible option. A life lived assuming all headaches are a brain tumor would be tough. *Believe me.* I've picked my daughter up from her school's infirmary with a headache, vomiting, and lethargy and took her directly to the MRI myself and scanned her, convinced it was a brain tumor until it was not.

"I'm sorry," I told them, looking directly at the father, who was tearing up. "This is not the time for the longer story. If we are going to get her legs working again, then I need you to sign the consent form and I need to go now. We will do our very best. I promise."

They signed the form and I left them at the main OR door silently staring at us all the way until we turned the corner to go into the room.

In the OR we found a tight clot of blood just underneath the laminae of several thoracic vertebrae. The compression was significant. Once the bone came off, the dura pushed the clot up off the spinal cord underneath, trying to spring back to a normal anatomical position. We saw two large arteries entering just above and below the clot—"pipes," we call them, as in "Hoo-boy, look at those pipes . . . be careful"—so we coagulated and cut those just before taking the whole clot out en masse and sending it for path. I saw no obvious tumor, the most common thing to be compressing a three-year-old's spine and causing them not to be able to walk.

"Well, that's a good thing," I remarked under my breath.

I briefly spoke to the family on the way out around 2:00 A.M. and assured them that "it may take a few days before we know, but we will be doing all that we can in the meantime," which is a bit of the neurosurgeon's mantra after emergency surgery such as this, particularly in the wee hours.

I made it back to sleep until, at 5:00 A.M., I was awakened by the resident's text that she was moving her toes. There was a little fist bump emoji next to the news. I sent one back and rolled over for a few more minutes of sleep.

By the time I was there at her bedside just before my first scheduled case of the day, she was lifting her legs up off the bed. The parents cried. The nurse cried. The resident and I cried a little too, she at the beginning of her career and me twenty years in, plus training. Both tired from the night's work but profoundly moved nonetheless. The short little toes wiggling and pudgy legs kicking the covers off the bed when hours before there was no movement whatsoever was pure joy.

The Peripheral Nervous System

In the cervical spine, several nerve roots peel off to exit the spinal cord to travel through lateral holes between the bones of the spinal column called the neural foramen, to combine and form the brachial plexus. This plexus of nerves jumbles up, amazingly in a predictable way, over the next several centimeters until five main nerves are formed that innervate the main muscle of the arm. These five main nerves are as critical to effecting movement of the arm as all the other parts of the chain in the central nervous system. A similar pattern to the nerves also occurs in the lower spine. The lumbosacral plexus forms from the nerves to and from the legs and pelvic structures. All critical for locomotion, bladder and bowel continence, and sexual function. A severe enough injury along either the brachial or the lumbosacral plexus, or related nerves, can shut the whole communication chain down, just like anywhere else. The recovery potential in the peripheral nervous system, however, as we will see later, is much more promising than with the spinal cord.

BACK NOW TO that ongoing operation where you are poised over the brain's surface. You've already opened the dura, swung in the scope, and glimpsed the brain underneath, the rolling patterns of the gyri and sulci along the surface, pulsing red arteries and laconic blue veins traveling mostly in pairs in and out and up and down. The clear CSF spills out around your instruments as you open. It is wondrous and you are still awed by its beauty.

Yet over there just off the midline, you can see a slight bulging of the brain, the gyri is expanded just barely, the vessels slightly more spaced out from one another in that area. You've carefully opened the surface. You use a sterile ultrasound probe to confirm. Just there! On the screen a shaggy white ball—the tumor—lies a few centimeters under the surface. When you see it, you are reminded that you are there not to be mesmerized but to act, to excise the invader, and then to retreat with as little impact on the human being beneath these drapes as possible.

"Bipolar in the left hand, sucker in the right," you say quietly each and every time you are poised over the precipice. From the next point onward, there is no going back.

The scrub tech hands them both directly to your outstretched hands without your having to look away from your target. With gentle motions of the sucker you advance a path through the surface gray matter deeper into the white matter. A minute later, you've yet to see the tumor where you expected. *How deep is this thing again?* you wonder. Your heart begins to beat a little faster, the tiniest bead of sweat forms on your forehead as your autonomic nervous system kicks in. *I'm certain we are well away from the motor strip, right? I measured three times on the MRI.* You gingerly advance another five millimeters deeper.

Then, suddenly, with the gentlest of swipes the glistening creamy white of the brain gives way to the dark edge of tumor, just there, just underneath the tips of your instruments. Under the microscope you can see the vivid contrast between the light and the dark.

Hovering, just for a span of a breath, the briefest of moments, you take in the enormousness of where you are and what you intend to do. Then, like all the times before, you begin.

4

Ninety Minutes from You by Ground

O N   A   B L U S T E R Y, rainy Saturday, in my first year of practice, I went to my office after rounds, put my feet up on my desk, took a sip of lukewarm coffee, and leaned back in my chair to relax after a busy morning. Within seconds, I felt the pager clipped to my belt vibrate. I set my mug down on the desk and called the number back. An emergency room doctor from another hospital immediately picked up and identified himself.

"Doc," said a clipped voice, "we've got a nine-year-old girl who was a rear passenger in a two-car collision about two hours ago. She's just arrived. The scan shows a three-centimeter subdural hematoma on the right side of her brain. We're a small show. Can you take her?"

"Yes," I said immediately. "What's her exam?"

"Her right pupil is blown, and she's posturing on the left."

The pupil typically dilates on the side of the brain with the increased pressure, in this case the right side, as the brain is forced down and away from the blood clot. The nerve responsible for pupillary function basically goes haywire and starts to enlarge in response. The term "posturing" describes a movement pattern that comes from damage being done to the part of the brain that deals with movement. Both are outward signs of high brain pressure. Put bluntly, this girl was sick, getting sicker quickly, and the window to save her was closing.

"Why don't you already have her in the air?" I asked, slightly annoyed. My hospital was in Birmingham, Alabama; theirs was in Auburn, a hundred miles away. A medical helicopter could have her here in just over thirty minutes, well within the window to save her.

"Weather's too bad between Auburn and Birmingham to fly in. She's ninety minutes from you by ground, at least," he said, clearly knowing what that meant—an hour and a half in an ambulance, plus the two hours since her accident, is a long time to have high intracranial pressure and expect to survive.

"What do we do?" he asked.

Even now, when I'm faced with a situation without an obvious solution, my mind goes to my father and the calmness I felt flying next to him as a child. During his more than four decades of service in the Air National Guard, he piloted all types of planes in all types of situations and weather. Early on, he taught me to review the flight checklist before every takeoff and landing. Once aloft, we would practice emergencies in the air. As we would gain altitude, and I would be focused on keeping the plane level on the horizon or interpreting the navigation system, he would quietly feather the propellers the tiniest amount, or trim the flaps just so. Then, as we gently lost airspeed and the altimeter would slowly begin to wind down under his watchful eye, he would have me "work the problem" until I had it figured out. Flying and problem solving for him went hand in hand and were as much a part of him as breathing.

As the brief memory faded, I found myself staring at the worn photo of him that sat on my office desk. He is standing next to an F-4 Phantom, helmet under his arm, grinning widely in his olive-drab National Guard flight suit.

"Are those Black Hawk helicopters still stationed at that base near you?" I asked the emergency room doctor.

"Yes, but . . ." He trailed off. Then he was back: "Yes! Those guys will fly in anything."

"You get the Black Hawks. I'll let our operating room know."

My office overlooked the street in front of the hospital. After half an hour, I looked down to see the surface of the coffee in my mug rippling like in the scene in *Jurassic Park* where the approaching *T. rex*'s footsteps are detected in puddles of water. Within seconds, there were rhythmic pulsations all around, then a strong thump-thump-thump-thump as the air beat against my window. Outside in the midst of the downpour, trash cans tumbled down the street and pickup trucks were forced down on their shocks. I gazed up to see an army Black Hawk helicopter, giant in comparison to our standard medical helicopters, hovering steadily over the children's hospital helipad, rain and fog swirling in all directions. Every part of the office thumped, the heartbeat in my own chest now overpowered.

Events moved quickly after the girl's arrival. In the pediatric trauma bay, two of the soldiers who brought her through the storm, still in their wet flight gear, worked alongside our nurses. As I came to the bedside, one of the nurses greeted me by name, and the younger of the two soldiers for some inexplicable reason immediately snapped to attention.

A vision of my father in his flight suit flashed in my head.

"At ease, soldier," I said. "I should be saluting you."

As we packaged the child up and headed off to the elevator up to the operating room, I turned back to them. There they stood amid the residual chaos of the trauma room, torn paper packaging and discarded blue gowns strewn about. They watched us roll into the elevator. I locked eyes with the closest soldier. He gave the briefest of nods just before the doors closed. Then he and the chaos of the trauma bay were gone.

The OR team was ready for her, the sterile instruments laid out on the back tables, blue drapes applied after a quick clipping of her hair and lightning-fast wash of her head with sterilizing prep solution. In lifesaving operations like this, as the clock has ticked past zero, the typical precision of neurosurgery loses out to speed. Speed at all costs. *Knife. No, damn it, we can stop the skin bleeding later.*

Retractor. Drill. Scissors to open the dura, bulging and tight from the underlying blood. The liquid part of the clot jets out around the scissors as we cut. Once the brain is exposed, it does the work for us, extruding most of the solid coagulated clot out in a matter of seconds. We clean out what is left at the edges, and I see the offending vein, torn away from the brain during the accident. We coagulate it and begin to make our way out, step by step, gently repairing all that we had to take apart to get there.

After surgery, she immediately began to stabilize, waking up and even flickering her eyes open, but her recovery took time and her journey was not without cost. She was left with a noticeable weakness on the left side and the slightest slur to her speech, but she was alive. With each follow-up appointment, some hurdle had been overcome. Over time, I would receive updates from her family. She would come to enter and then win a local beauty and talent pageant; be voted Most School Spirit; cheer alongside friends dressed up as the school mascot; and then, one remarkable May day, graduate from high school. Four years later, she would finish college and head to graduate school for a career in social work. All of this chronicled first in clinic visits, then, as the medical reasons to see me faded, in holiday cards and the occasional letter.

A decade and a half after her injury I received one such letter. No longer the hand-drawn cards of childhood or newspaper clippings from her proud parents, this was a handwritten note on elegant stationery inviting me to her wedding. *Her wedding.* I could still see her in the bed of the pediatric ICU after surgery—a nine-year-old child with abrasions on the side of her face from the accident and a clean white head wrap around her head. The nurses methodically connecting her to the monitors, line by line, tube by tube. Me urging her to squeeze my hand, for a sign, any sign, that she was better. Now, years later, I was reading how thankful she was to have been given this chance. Grateful for those soldiers in that helicopter, for the two hospital teams, and for me. She promised to always have us in mind as she began her new married life and hopefully one day raised her own family.

As I read the letter sitting in a different office in a different city, thinking back over those events, I found myself realizing how deeply grateful I was for her evolving story over the years—all the cards, each barrier broken, every milestone—and for what that experience taught me. So many other critically ill children in the subsequent years benefited from this early experience, when I was learning how hard to push, where to draw the line, and how much to expect of others.

My father's lessons in the air, that industrious emergency room doctor, those brave soldiers soaked to the bone standing there as we rolled away—so many people and events came together for this one child to grow into her life, to find happiness, to find love. All of us need a living, breathing reminder to just keep pushing on. There may be a life there to be beautifully and fully lived, a person who just needs someone, anyone, to work the problem, to make the hard call, and to fly in a storm.

5

We Have a Protocol for That

THERE WERE TIMES during my neurosurgical residency that shook to the foundation who I believed myself to be and then over time fundamentally altered who I actually was. As those long blurred-together years in training passed, we were hardened, the ability to connect on a meaningful level with our patients, and even each other over time, nearly purged from us by necessity, as a means of self-protection. Certainly there were many saves and successes along the way; I'm not sure anyone could finish a six- or seven-year neurosurgery residency if there were not. But what I tend to remember from my training are not the days in which we operated on four patients in a row with brain tumors, each one awakening better off than when they went under, or the grateful sixty-year-old veteran with, for the first time in five years, resolved back pain after spine surgery, or even the first aneurysm I ever clipped, a supposed rite of passage as a neurosurgery resident. The times I remember the most are the times I first felt that heavy weight of responsibility. When the magnitude of that broke through whatever protective shell I had formed. It was not long into my training that I found out that my actions or inactions, or even brief hesitations, could save a life or lose a life. Just like that.

I remember trying to pull the woman's bed out of the ICU myself. Her pupils were fixed and dilated; she had only the smallest amount of brainstem function left. Thirty minutes before, she was on the ward and talking, being worked up for a vague dizziness that came on and off over the previous few days. Within a matter of seconds, her entire exam went to hell. She was scanned and sent to the medical ICU because there were no beds in the neuro-ICU, the typical unit for acute stroke patients. As the neurosurgery resident on call, I took the consult and ran upstairs to see her just after the head CT was performed. After a quick exam, I called my attending to recount her story. The general gist: cerebellar stroke, actively herniating. Close to death. Her only chance was surgery to remove the overlying bone—a decompression. The skull that had protected her during life was now constricting her brain as it swelled, tighter and tighter. The pressure inside her head could be tolerated for only so long.

"Get her down to the OR now," he said matter-of-factly. "Bring her yourself."

I ran back over to her room and told the team around her what I had just been told.

"Well, we have to have respiratory therapy come," one said.

"The patient is not even admitted to the ICU yet," said another.

"We've got to go now," I said, starting to pull the bed free and roll the IV pole with her. "Somebody start bagging her for transport."

"Stop right now! Who do you think you are?" someone yelled.

"She's going to die," I shouted back.

"Cut the theatrics; we have a protocol."

I kept trying to pull her away. The respiratory therapist was busy and couldn't come over to help. The nurse refused to let me take her. The charge nurse stepped in and threatened to call my attending. I begged her to.

This went on for twenty minutes, the back-and-forth, the tug-of-war. Me pulling the bed out a foot, the nurses yelling for me to stop. Me yelling out for the respiratory therapist to come help.

Then my attending appeared in the door. He walked over and examined her. Her brainstem reflexes had gone. She had progressed to brain death.

He looked at me, eyes blazing.

"I told you to get her to the OR," he said.

"I tried, sir." I looked down at the floor as I said it.

"She's dead," he said. "She's dead and her only chance was you."

With that he looked around the room at everyone standing there frozen. He peered directly into the eyes of each person, one by one, and paused for just a moment. Then, just as quickly as he entered, he walked out. Soon everyone filed out of the room quietly.

She had a sudden stroke of one side of her cerebellum and had herniated, basically the brain at the base of the skull swelling so much that it pushes out the bottom of the skull. That kind of pressure, sustained for too long, results in brain death more often than not. An operation to remove part of the skull and the part of the brain that had stroked would have taken under two hours to do, skin to skin. It could have brought her back.

Years have gone by since she died. I don't remember interacting with anyone in that unit again during my residency. In truth, over the next three years, I avoided it at all costs. I wonder if any of them who were there think of that time. I think of it a good bit. Some neurosurgeons would say that she had little chance of survival, her exam too gone for surgery to have had an impact. But trying to justify her death by saying that it wouldn't have mattered seems like a cheap out to me, even with two decades of experience since then. Perhaps it is *because* of two decades of experience since then. If my family had a 15 percent chance, would I take it? Ten percent? Five percent? Five percent is one in twenty. I have taken those odds before; many of us in pediatric neurosurgery have. And I have seen children and young adults come back. Recover to the point of having a purpose in life and to love and be loved.

My attending knew that by placing the blame on me, by pointing his vitriol at me, he would be indirectly placing it on everyone involved and that they would know. Then the next time a patient needed to go to the OR emergently in this ICU where patients rarely had neurosurgical issues, there would be no hesitation on anyone's part. It's taken me some time, and years of training residents, to have some understanding of that day. But I get it now. The effect on me? It's driven me in times when I felt the system wasn't moving fast enough. I've ripped off the monitors and carried a child acutely ill up from the emergency room myself, past the excuses and the process and the red tape, into the OR so that we could fix their failing ventricular shunt. I'm not particularly proud of that, but it was necessary. I have also defended a resident for doing the same to get a middle-aged woman having a stroke up to the angiogram suite for treatment. She walked out intact the next day. That I am indeed proud of.

For this woman, this experience, I fall back to this unresolved time. One where I cannot change the outcome, only replay it in my head. I remember standing in the hall as her family filed in to say goodbye. I faced each one as they walked by, some looking at me. Some not. I was convinced they knew that I had failed her, even though they were not there for the blaming. I remember the wail of her young daughter as she turned into the room to see her mother, now and forever gone. I can still hear it, still know that feeling that everything on this earth was channeling through my chest at that moment and how I wanted to wink out of existence, never to return.

An hour later, I scrubbed in with that same attending. We were operating on a thirty-five-year-old with a sizable AVM in the right temporal lobe. Our hands moved in unison under the microscope, carefully separating the tangle of blood vessels from the surrounding normal brain. Then, suddenly, a flash of bright red blood—

a feeding vessel had torn free. The blood welled up in the field. The brain began to swell. We placed our surgical suckers in the cavity blindly and after several more seconds found the source. I put a single clip across it, and the bleeding stopped.

"Nice job," he said.

6

———•◦•———

GSW to Head

I N T H E S P R I N G of my fifteenth year of practice, I found myself looking down at a three-year-old reaching around blindly with his right arm as his sedation began to wear off. His left arm lay at his side, unmoving. A large wad of gauze, placed in haste by the ambulance medics, was held against the right side of his head by a loose, bloody head wrap. Underneath, a fist-sized area of skin and skull was missing. His right pupil was larger than his left, a sign of brain pressure, but still reacting to light because the normally constraining box of the skull had been blown open by the bullet passing through.

The familiar movement of resuscitation flowed around me as the breathing tube was secured and intravenous lines were placed urgently. There was coagulated blood everywhere, pooling under his head and dripping down like candle wax onto the floor. A track of bloody footprints grew larger and larger as the crowd gathered around him, coming and going with bulging IV bags of blood or saline and syringes of medication to try to stabilize the blood pressure.

The charge nurse standing near a desk outside the room said, "Neurosurgery, it's the OR calling for you. Are we coming now?"

"We are coming right now," someone said. The voice was mine. "Do we know where the parents are?"

*   *   *

SOON WE ARE in the OR. The chaos follows us the whole way.

"We're hanging trauma blood," said Tom, a longtime anesthesia colleague. "And we need every inch below the neck if we can have it." Trauma blood was stockpiled in refrigerators nearby for emergencies when there was no time to wait for a cross match. O negative is the universal donor and least likely to start up a transfusion reaction, a possibly lethal cascade when the body rejects the blood being given.

"I'll prep. Let's take just the head," I said to the surgical team. "Bring the poles all the way up here."

In the most urgent cases, our anesthesia colleagues will keep placing lines, or adjusting flow, or a multitude of *whatever the hell they need to do to keep the kid alive.* In such cases, instead of an orderly prepping and draping where each and every piece of equipment is carefully put just so—surgical cautery on the right, suctions just off to both sides, the drill on the left with the pedal that controls the speed under my right foot—we basically throw prep on the wound as fast as we can, towel it out, and drape only the top of the head, sparing the face as well as the rest of the body. In our haste, all the cords and wires going to the cautery, the suction, the drill, everything quickly becomes a jumbled mess.

Tom speaks up: "His pressure is tanking." Tom is that experienced, unflappable anesthesiologist who has seen patients and surgeons come and go here for a while. When he's in my room, I don't even have to think about their side of the drapes. "We can't keep up," he says. "You'd better stop the bleeding now." Coming from Tom, that is bad. About-to-die bad.

I looked down to the mishmash below me. Hundreds of tiny blood vessels on the surface of the brain were disrupted and bleeding. The dura was ripped open all the way to the skull edge, nearly to the midline sagittal sinus. The sagittal sinus is a triangular-shaped flume that drains nearly all of the blood of the brain. When this is torn or disrupted in any way, particularly in a child, you have to handle it quickly, or, depending on the age, the child exsanguinates—dies from blood loss. Fortunately for this one, *finally something fortunate,* the sinus was intact, and I had no intention of wandering too close to change that. Blood oozed from the bone edges in spots. *We can wax that.* Bone wax is exactly what it sounds like, sterilized wax that can be pressed into the bone and stops the blood coming from the vascular cancellous bone that runs inside the inner and outer table of the jagged bone edge. The most rapid blood loss in front of us, however, came from the torn skin edges. The scalp has an intricate maze of blood vessels that keep it nourished and healthy. This is why when you cut your head, it bleeds profusely. Scalp bleeding from a straight or smaller cut will usually stop with direct pressure, but here the severed ends of multiple scalp arteries that run just underneath the layer of protective fat in the scalp are pulsing away, adding to the growing pool of blood.

All of this takes about two seconds to take in.

And then we begin.

"We start on the skin and work our way in," I say to the third-year resident as I place a surgical sponge directly down on the raw exposed and disrupted surface of the brain, a pack-it-off maneuver that slows even the worst bleeding. This has been done for years by surgeons and war medics all over the world in all sorts of conflicts, and in all parts of the body, including the sacred brain when you have to.

"Do what I do," I say to her. "And anticipate the next steps."

In academic surgery—surgery practiced at a high-volume referral center where both education and research are also valued—residents are critical to the mission. In exchange for the opportunity to learn the craft of neurosurgery, the residents take first call, handle much of the nonsensical extra work piled upon us by the electronic medical record, and keep the trains running. Each operation is "covered" by a resident, meaning a resident is assigned to assist in that case. Depending on the experience level (and difficulty of the case and number of cases for the day and so on), the resident will have various levels of involvement. In private practice there is a trained first assist, or on occasion one's partner will assist if necessary. In academics, it's always a resident. I've never known anything else but academic neurosurgery, and I cannot imagine not having a trainee by my side. In my world, operating and teaching go hand in hand. I am aware that there are much better teachers than me, and that the residents oftentimes like a teaching style less influenced by a more dogmatic bygone era, but one of the things that I am most proud of is the number of adult and pediatric neurosurgeons out there whom I have had at least a small modicum of influence on. I certainly have been influenced myself along the way, both by the attending surgeons who have taught me and by the resident surgeons I have had the opportunity to train.

Quickly cauterizing the bleeding ends of the scalp vessels one by one and placing specially designed plastic clips across the skin edges designed to compress vessels and stop bleeding after scalp incisions, we pick tiny splinters of skull out from seemingly everywhere as we go. The resident places two retractors that hold the skin edges back and expose the area where the real operation is about to begin. *Attagirl,* I think, careful not to speak out loud. It would have been a verbal "attaboy" had the resident been a male, but we must be careful about any perception of condescension with trainees nowadays, male or female.

Recently, the number of women entering surgery has increased substantially. While not quite as much as in other surgical fields, that increase holds across North American neurosurgical programs as well, reaching up to 15 percent in the last several years. At one point during my years directing the neurosurgical training program here at Vanderbilt, six of nineteen neurosurgery residents were women. I've had the opportunity to mentor all of them in some way, and they are finding their way into every subspecialty within our field. Women have been a welcome addition to the field of neurosurgery, but they have had to fight to get here. Men had had the monopoly for quite long enough, and the training and culture had gotten too malignant, too testosterone-driven. I'm not saying that women can't be tough. I've known plenty of them tougher than me. But I also have been influenced by one mother, two sisters, a wife, and a daughter, and if I did not come out of those experiences realizing that those viewpoints are as valid as mine, then I have wasted the opportunity.

"Attagirl," I say. To heck with it. She needs the same feedback to keep making good aggressive decisions. Emboldened, she picks up the drill.

"Now the bone." We take the drill and remove chunks of fragmented skull from around the edges, carefully beginning to sculpt out an oval-shaped defect that will enable a skull implant to fit better in the future, when we bring him back to fix the defect. *If he survives this*. After we wax the bone edges, things do start to calm down a little. We still have direct pressure on the brain surface, holding the multitude of disrupted vessels at bay, for the moment. For the first time since we put them up, I look over the surgical drapes to see Tom and the team pulling blood out of the IV bags and forcibly injecting it into our patient. They are desperately trying to get blood back into him to get his pressure up.

"Forty over ten," he yells out. "Do you have control of that bleeding yet?"

"Yes," I quickly answer. "We're at a holding point for now. Go ahead and catch up and let me know when I can keep going." This running dialogue between surgeon and anesthesiologist is crucial, particularly in high-intensity situations like this, where there is no opportunity for a do-over. If I as a surgeon create a culture where the anesthesia team, be it doctor or nurse anesthetist, does not feel comfortable to speak up when things are going south, then that is my fault, not theirs. Communication is key. Knowing when a patient is about to code on the table is key. Knowing it way before they actually do is ideal for the very reason that we may be able to do something to avoid it.

As we more gently now hold pressure with the gauze on the exposed surface of the brain, I watch Tom and the team stabilize the blood pressure with trauma blood and other concentrated blood products which help to reverse any blood thinning, and lack of clotting, that can occur with multiple transfusions. The blood pressure begins to rise and the heart rate, dangerously high only a few minutes ago, begins to come down closer to normal. Low blood pressure and a high heart rate happen as a physiological result of hemorrhagic shock, when blood loss is perilously high. With circulating blood volume at critically low levels, the heart pumps faster to try to make up the difference. This type of shock is way more common in general or thoracic surgery trauma, where bullets or motor vehicle collisions tear open major internal blood vessels and the patient starts to bleed out. In truth, the vast majority of people who have a gunshot wound to the head die either at the scene or soon after arrival.

"We're better," says Tom, interrupting my thoughts on the next few steps. "Go for it."

The resident and I meticulously work together in a clockwise fashion and pick off each of the bleeding brain blood vessels one by one, either with the surgical cautery or with tiny little titanium vascular clips. We find the dural edge and sew a large patch all the way around the defect in the dura with the idea of trying to keep cerebrospinal fluid from leaking out of the wound after surgery, inviting infection and leading to meningitis.

Today is not the day to worry about the open bone defect. A large piece of his own skull is gone, and what's left is not directly repairable today. The risk of infection is too great. We can come back another day and place a sterile 3-D-printed replacement graft specifically designed to fit perfectly based on a special thin-slice CT template. This technology has come a long way from the times of taking sterile methyl methacrylate—also known as bone cement—pouring it into the defect, the smell nearly overwhelming, and irrigating quickly to reduce the chance of burning the dura or brain from the thermogenic—that is, really hot—reaction as the cement sets. The extra bits of dried cement would be drilled off and come to cover the surgical field in a granular mess until irrigated away. All of this effort made for a moderately well-fitting implant at best. The difference now is at least an hour less in the OR, a significantly better fit, and a much neater surgical field. I also suspect much less particulate matter inhaled into all of our lungs, too.

Looking down, now we must focus on getting the skin closed, no small task because of the blast effect where a portion was blown away. Taking lessons from past plastic surgery colleagues, we extend our incision along the back of the head about an inch and a half and curve slightly toward the back of the ear so that we can bring the more lateral skin flap forward and make up for the destroyed or unusable skin. We then undermine the normal skin by loosening it from the underlying bone in order to mobilize it for closure, rotate the side of the scalp forward, and place a series of heavy interrupted sutures, like thick fishing line, that serve to bring the skin edges together. A drain under the skin will help to remove fluid and allow the edges to heal. The area on the forehead above the right eye, right where the bullet entered, is a hole, the plug of skin long gone. We can cut back the ragged edges, but ultimately we just have to place ungraceful heavy sutures across it and hope it holds. The resident quickly places an intracranial pressure monitor, a one-millimeter wire, in the brain on the opposite side of the head before we roll up to the pediatric intensive care unit. This tiny wire measures the pressure inside the head after surgery and helps to guide therapy in the roller-coaster critical days after surgery.

"Strong work, everyone." I say this looking directly at the scrub nurse, who I realize did a terrific job of keeping up and whom I had never worked with before. She smiles.

"Way more exciting than urology," she deadpans.

TWO WEEKS LATER, we are dangling a stuffed tiger over the bed. The boy reaches up with his right hand and swats at it, squealing with frustration if we start to take it away. His left arm lies by his side. He laughs as we make the tiger appear over the bed rail and pretend to stalk him. He has a feeding tube entering through his nose, but not for much longer. We've watched him eat a little cereal while we are in the room. Spider-Man figurines lie in the bed next to him, on his right side only.

Soon he and his family will transition to a pediatric rehabilitation facility so that he can undergo weeks of dedicated therapy designed to strengthen his left side rendered weak from the damage to the right side of the brain caused by the bullet. It will help. In probably three months or so, he will return for the skull implant. What life will he go back to? What job will he hold one day? Now at three years old, he will forever know no other reality than this, the story of the jagged scar on the side of his head.

I walk back to the door of his hospital room and lean against the frame, watching the therapists use toys to motivate him to interact and show the family how to gently push him in between sessions. Why did this particular child survive when so many do not? Not every person with a gunshot wound to the head makes it to the OR. If the bullet passes across the midline of the brain or involves the CSF spaces inside the brain or crosses the brainstem where the housekeeping functions of the brain happen, where the heartbeat, breathing, and level of awareness are held, then typically no surgery can help them. For this boy, the path of the bullet both permanently disabled him and, oddly, saved him. The fact that the skull had been blown open, on one side only, the nondominant right side—where no speech function resides—allowed the pressure to go out, not in. This, and a system that got him to the OR quickly, made all the difference.

My mind drifts back to a long-ago head wrap, tight on the head of a thirty-year-old who had just arrived by ambulance. "GSW to head in ED" had appeared on my pager, and I, as the on-call third-year neurosurgery resident, was already in the ED seeing an endless series of consults. A surgical clamp poked up through the folds of the wrap, pulsing with every heartbeat. Nobody in the ED wanted to touch it. I cut through layer after layer of bloody gauze until I found that the hemostat was clamped across multiple large branches of the left middle cerebral artery, a major blood vessel supplying a large swath of his brain on the left, which had been torn open along with brain and a large part of the skull by the short-range shotgun blast earlier that evening. In addition to right-sided function, the left side—the dominant hemisphere—is where language and the ability to communicate reside. Without those, we are hostages in the world, unable to interact in a meaningful way.

As we ran his stretcher to the elevator that led directly to the OR, his right side lay still, his eyes were closed, only garbled sounds coming from his mouth. His speech area was destroyed with no chance of recovery. He survived thanks to that surgery and the quick thinking of whoever initially applied that clamp. He would never, however, walk or talk again. That day in the OR as we started the operation, my attending said to me, *Do what I do. Anticipate the next steps. Attaboy.* I remember placing the retractors, taking up the drill, stopping the bleeding. Working with my attending. Step by step.

As I stand there thinking about that day, it becomes clear to me that these two patients are forever linked. Both gunshot wounds to the head. Both unnecessary events with lifelong consequences. Both pulled back from just over the edge. The difference, however, was critical. The thirty-year-old mute man had his life devastated by the injury. He would never interact with society again. The three-year-old playing in the bed was a different story. The two were separated by the centimeters of a different bullet trajectory, and that distance could have been miles.

There in his room I am mesmerized by his facial expressions. He blinks as he looks directly at the therapist as the meaning of her words clearly begins to register. I see him look out past us into the hall as one of the therapists holds out her hand for a high five.

"KJ," he says, turning to focus on her and reaching up to match his good hand to hers. "My name is KJ."

7

Family Charades

Years before I was born, when my sisters, Eve and Sarah, were eight and four years old and living with my parents in Richmond, Virginia, our father brought home a new color television set for Christmas. A huge thing, as deep as it was wide, with a rotary knob for twelve channels. I imagine the weight of it being nearly overbearing. After cajoling a work friend to help and then struggling to bring it in one afternoon while the girls were away, Dad found it to fit neatly under a table near the far corner of the den. The floor-length tablecloth, he thought, would be all that was needed to complete the camouflage for the three weeks prior to Christmas.

Dad's perspective, however, was from the vantage of an adult walking past or sitting in the room to read the newspaper or talk with friends. He failed to consider the perspective of two children who skipped and tumbled and crawled in and around things. The afternoon after the TV had been hidden, four-year-old Sarah began to crawl under her favorite hiding spot from her sister when she hit her head on something solid. She lifted up the edge of the cloth and, realizing what she had discovered, excitedly ran into the kitchen to let Eve in on her newfound knowledge. Mom, overhearing and acting fast, bargained with them, allowing one hour of TV-watching each day as long as Dad was never told that they knew of the surprise. Henceforth, every weekday around 3:30, once Eve came home from school, the girls would lift up the tablecloth and watch one hour of children's afternoon television before Dad came home. Mom must have felt a mix of emotions ranging from 1960s housewife guilt to being quite tickled about her crisis avoidance and negotiation skills with her two young daughters.

One night, after the girls had gone to bed, Dad decided that they had been asleep long enough and that he and Mom could watch some of the new color TV he had brought home. He carefully cracked the door to the girls' room to confirm they were sound asleep in their twin beds, then quietly closed it, putting towels along the bottom of the door to keep the sound from disturbing them. Mom took all this in, realizing that she was now a double agent in her own home. Soon there she was, stealing moments of TV by day with the girls and by night with my father. Day after day. Night after night. Navigating, somehow, through all of it, keeping both sides' secrets.

With one week left until Christmas, Dad mentioned to a small group of neighbors that he had gotten his family a color TV and was excited to pull off his grand surprise. The issue of course was that Eve had already told her neighborhood friends, who told their mothers, who told their husbands. Nearly the whole block knew that his family spent the afternoon watching the new TV that he had so carefully hidden under the table in the den. They egged him on to tell the story in front of other friends over and over until the story of John and his new color TV was the neighborhood story of that year's Christmas. When Christmas Day finally did come, no one was happier than my mother, exhausted from living this double life. The children, having rehearsed a mock unveiling ahead of time with her, held hands and jumped up and down when the TV was unveiled, joyously hugging Dad and Mom, playing their parts perfectly.

The exact time when Dad actually found out the truth was lost to family lore with the passing of my mother years after his own death. Perhaps it happened just after the unveiling, revealed by my sisters or Mom or a co-worker, or much later in life around the family table. It is uncertain to me if he ever actually knew the full story of Mom's role, or his friends', or if it even matters that these small untruths or narratives that we create are ever really supposed to be revealed.

My aunt Robin, my mother's younger sister, harbored wonderful memories of visiting cousins in Gig Harbor, Washington, as a young child. This branch of the family was linked to ours through Mom and Robin's father, Chuck, and his two larger-than-life brothers who settled down there when the family separated after years in Northern California. My grandfather followed a successful athletic career at Stanford with a job as an assistant coach on the University of Mississippi football team. The other two Smalling boys made their way to Washington State and settled there, marrying and starting families. A generation later came the wonderfully gregarious cousin Jay Smalling, who over time came to know the perfect joke for every occasion and the rules to nearly every card game in existence. Jay was eternally kind and loving, my own mother's favorite cousin, who had a delightful mischievous streak that bubbled just under the surface, like his father. And like his own son would have one day. With a distant mother, busy father, and sister separated by more than a decade in age, my mother came to see Jay as a brother figure. Years later, when I came into the family, I was initially named after my father, who himself was a junior. She would come to persuade my father to nickname their only son, me, after Jay when the realization that two Johns in the household was more complicated than they were willing to endure. I have come to believe that this was Mom's intention the entire time, never knowing the havoc to be wreaked to my frequent-flier account in the years to come.

Jay and his wife, Peachy, had two children themselves and were constantly entertaining in their home on the water of Puget Sound with a dock house full of skiffs, ski boats, sailboats, and rowers and their very own pickleball court built into the hill above their home. Into one particular late summer many years ago came my aunt Robin, visiting as a seven-year-old with her parents, and without my mother, who was in college at the time. One day, the Puget Sound Smalling family persuaded Robin to fish off their dock, and true to form, Jay secretly snuck under the dock and hooked Robin's line with a tremendous store-bought salmon. He then gave the line two quick tugs for good measure. Unaware, seven-year-old Robin proceeded to call out to everyone that she had a bite, then squeal with delight and reel in what would reveal itself to be a giant fish that would in time take on mythic proportions. The fact that the fish was dead and cold made no impact on her. It was the bending of the pole, the excitement of her family around her, and the sheer joy of reeling in a fish that sealed in the memory.

In Robin's case, it was nearly fifty years later, in our family's southern Mississippi home during a winter's holiday lunch surrounded by family that she finally heard the truth. I sat directly across from her as it unfolded. Told casually by someone at the table, as if she already knew, the story was followed by laughter and happiness all around. I watched as Robin, whitening slightly, became still and quiet, tightly gripping a small tissue in her lap. She quickly righted, admitting with a chuckle that she had never known. *Oh that cousin Jay Smalling, wasn't he something.* Soon enough, the conversation moved on.

Later, after the dishes were cleared and the silver sat soaking in the bottom of the sink, I watched her walk to the far corner of our backyard. Well past the line of towering jagged pecan trees and the thicket of camellias in full winter bloom. There, overlooking the wild rows of the fallow garden, she stood for a long while in the late afternoon shadows. I imagine her thinking through that childhood memory for the last time, loving it, then letting it go.

Years later, Melissa and I lived in Jackson, Mississippi, as I finished up the final year of medical school. After nearly two years we had decided to no longer put off the inevitable and became engaged. We invited my parents out for a celebratory lunch, and with glasses raised, we announced our intention to marry. Mirth and happiness abounded. We toasted our family, our future, ourselves. Soon with my father's happy announcement to all that could hear, the entire restaurant joined in and did the same. I then, in what I have come to see as my last act of childhood innocence, turned to my father and asked if he would be the best man in our wedding.

Other than that day, I rarely saw my father cry outright. I can see him sitting there in that booth. Bread on the table, a few crumbs littered around his bread plate. Salad fork perched in midair. *No fresh ground pepper, thank you,* as the waitress walks up and away quickly. Then, just in the moments as I was asking, I can see the change that washes across his face with realization, as emotion unexpectedly takes him. Throughout his life, my father was a man well known for a near-constant optimism, who espoused that you could chart your own destiny if you only believed that you could do it. Successful in business, striking out on his own into the retail world early, and successful in an entire second parallel life as a pilot of anything with fixed wings in the Air National Guard, he never wavered in his support and love for his children. As with many children and their parents, there was much left for me to understand in him. For that moment, however, announcing my impending marriage, I saw myself as taking a significant step out of a murky prolonged adolescence into adulthood with years ahead to grow with him and learn from him, one day settling into middle age with an elderly and proud father looking back on an accomplished life and loving family.

After the tearful yes, the pride of the day, the joy, I remember a simple conversation as we walked out of the restaurant before splitting up for the ride home. Dad took me aside and casually mentioned he had been having some recent weakness in his right hand. He first noticed it as he went to replace a coffee can on the top shelf of the refrigerator a few days earlier, when he lost his grip and the can tumbled to the ground and burst open. Flush in the joy of the day, I quickly made a promise to think through it better, perhaps asking some of my professors over in the medical school that Monday, not realizing at the time the significance of that moment.

Over months and numerous doctor visits, imaging, blood tests, and with me poring over medical texts and journals for an alternative diagnosis, this initial occasional grip weakness occurring only when the hand was held just so would reveal itself to be ALS, amyotrophic lateral sclerosis, a progressive and incurable neurodegenerative disease. The unending days now had an end. Unfathomable to me then, I would come to watch him lay down each aspect of his life: his flying, his driving, his work. Until all that was left was his breath, his family, his memories.

His death, however, would not come until eighteen months later. My parents were direct in their wishes to tell no one. Not friends, not family, and not my two older sisters. Initially, he could hide it by shrewd camouflage, no longer gesticulating during animated conversations or covering his hands with a jacket. Over time, however, it became obvious. Folks could see the gradual difficulty with writing and eating, but like the unwelcome guest everyone chooses to ignore at a party, the family charade was kept up. All of this was of course most worrisome to my sisters, whose concerned queries were answered with "We are seeing the doctor next week" or "A little physical therapy should clear this right up." This choice to stay in the present would later come to drive a slight, barely-present-but-there-like-a-splinter wedge between my sisters and me that would take time to heal and repair after Dad had died, when there was no one to blame and only sadness. I remember the days around the wedding itself, surrounded by friends and family, all joyous about our soon-to-be-new life and purposely refraining from any acknowledgment of my dad's illness. I have come to think often of that time when he stood next to me in front of the church, fumbled the ring out of his pocket with his barely moving fingers, and then looked into my face with pride and a need for forgiveness for all the past days lost while in the sky and those never to be had in the future. We would not grow older as father and son together. It would forever be as it was at his death, with me as a proto-adult just on the edge of understanding the mysteries of his life and his choices that were all beginning to unveil themselves to me as my own perspective changed. At that point all I knew was the anger at my inability to change the future rushing at us. It would be much later in my own life when I would feel near-desperate need of his wisdom, fumbling my own way through my life and work challenges, as I sought out other sources, re-creating over and over that relationship halted in time. Only to be left again with the emptiness and anger over his absence.

To my own son and daughter born more than a decade later, my father—the embodiment of courage and happiness, who lived a vibrant and idealized life to me as a boy that was now lost to me as a man—would be known only in stories told while sitting around the dining room table of that southern Mississippi family home at holidays. Over the years I brought my children to that home that for me represented nothing less than another dimension. One inhabited by my parents and me in my youth in the time after my sisters had left for college, in which the three of us coexisted together outside time. Later it was where I could collect and sustain the stories of my childhood and struggle through the forever unfinished life with my father.

In my own narrative, expunged of his later hospital bed, the intermittent mumbling, and the slowing of breath, he instead stands with me in that church on the cusp of a new life, my own life, and reaches into his breast pocket to proudly hand me the wedding ring. Raising his face up to mine, he brings a strong hand up to wipe away the sadness. Then after an embrace, he places my hands in my wife's and steps away. As I turn to face her, I last see him smiling, joyous, and striding away, fading forever into the hereafter.

8

Rubber Bands

"ARE THOSE RUBBER bands?" I asked myself incredulously. Standing there at the computer terminal at eye level in the middle of my busy clinic, I stared at a 3-D-reconstituted image on a computer screen. There, unmistakably, were two faint outlines, like tiny Möbius strips, looped back around themselves. Rubber bands. They were not supposed to be where I was seeing them.

FOR A REASON long lost to me, I have a small sense of pride in the fact that I use less expensive alternatives in the operating room when I can. Let me be clear here, though: neurosurgery overall is an expensive undertaking. The operating microscopes alone can be half a million dollars for hospitals to buy, intraoperative image-based navigation—like a GPS for operating—around the same. Both of those are near standard for most brain tumor resections these days.

But those are both also onetime charges that a hospital or medical system forks over in order for the surgeons to be able to take on the more complex cases with a higher degree of safety. (There is a story of a pediatric neurosurgeon from two generations ago who would just slightly bend his index finger, insert it into the interface between the tumor and normal cerebellum, and sweep the tumor up and out of the head. No microscope. No fancy instruments. Just his finger. Clearly, we have made progress since then as our expectations of neurologic outcomes and degree of tumor removal have evolved.) These types of "capital purchases"—microscopes, intra-operative navigation platforms, ultrasound probes—are not the same as day-to-day, case-to-case charges.

Nearly every operation requires trays and trays of sterilized equipment as well as disposable items, like gowns, gloves, and packets of sutures. Before COVID-19, most of us who worked in the OR went through multiple hats and surgical masks daily, never thinking twice about winding a mask up after you had worn it for a few minutes and tossing it into the trash. I think of some long-ago cartoon from childhood of a group of fat-cat types, rolling up hundred-dollar bills and lighting cigars with them. (This could also be an image captured in my memory from most MTV videos of the 1980s.) Clearly, this behavior has changed.

So, if I'm not talking about major equipment, OR trays, or even masks, then what am I talking about? Well, not infrequently, I use standard silk suture to secure the bone flap back to the skull instead of the more expensive absorbable or metal plates, particularly in infants whose skulls are thinner. It works great, the bone knits up just fine, and there is less than a dollar of additional cost compared with hundreds of times that. Another example: Instead of using the more expensive collagen dural substitute as a patch to close the dura as close to watertight as possible, I will carefully peel the patient's own pericranium off the surrounding skull surface and sew the paper-flat tissue into the defect, using the patient's own tissue as the patch. In certain situations, there is good data that doing that is superior to the alternatives. But make no mistake, I didn't make this stuff up. I was taught it by the generation of surgeons who influenced me.

Yet another example: After making the incision in the scalp, I will flap the skin back over a rolled-up sponge to keep a sharp angle from forming that could kink off the blood supply and cause the skin flap to die off. That part, just about everyone does. Instead of using disposable hooks to hold the skin flap back, though, I use a simple Vicryl suture and five-centimeter-long sterilized rubber bands to secure the tissue back out of the way. Easy. I've done hundreds of craniotomies this way, and I've never had a problem with the skin that I can remember. Once you see the results of poor technique, perhaps during training or in other surgeons' patients (of course, never your own, ahem), you never let those images go.

I've even taken out a subdural hematoma using a minor surgical tray (cue scrub nurse eye rolling), one that contains bare-bones instrumentation. Of course, it's possible I never did that, and maybe just by saying over and over for nearly twenty years that *I could take out a subdural hematoma* with such a tray, I have willed it into reality. All of this I know pales in comparison with my colleagues who operate in resource-limited parts of the world who reuse everything possible, including the plastic Raney clips used to stop skin bleeding or the old-fashioned non-powered hand drills and saws used to open the skull. The fact that surgery in the "developing" world has something to teach us in the "developed" world about conserving resources is not lost on me.

But regarding the taking-out-a-subdural-with-a-minor-tray part, I do think I keep this running concept in my mind as kind of a generalist pediatric neurosurgeon who could handle whatever is sent my way on call—a kind of *M*A*S*H*'s Hawkeye Pierce of pediatric neurosurgery, ready to take on whatever flies in by either fixing the problem or stabilizing things until someone else with more specific expertise comes along. I see myself with a cache of straightforward fixes, lots of "arrows in the quiver," I like to say. It's an important part of my identity. I think I am at my best when asked to handle diverse things well enough to get the job done and the patient cared for, and as often as possible really excel at something well enough to have a beautiful and life-restoring outcome.

And when the surgery is over, most of the instruments and disposables used need to be counted, to make sure that we have as much stuff once the operation is over as we had before it started. This process, as in much of what we do in medicine, is not foolproof. How urgent is the case? Is this an eight-year-old who has been hit on her bike and the surgical team is trying to stop the bleeding with anything they can get their hands on? Or is this an elective rhizotomy, a remarkable surgery done by one of my partners in which various sensory nerve roots are cut to help a child with cerebral palsy walk steadier, which is not at all under time pressure? Those are two very different environments. Add in fatigue, revolving personnel, and the fact that the surgery is being performed by a biped mammal who wears glasses and might not have had breakfast and there is not insignificant room for error.

So, now that the setting-the-stage, justification-of-my-ways part is done, I can more easily admit that over the course of my surgical life and thousands of operations on children, I have managed to join the ignoble ranks of surgeons who have inadvertently left an object in a patient, an event otherwise known as a "retained foreign body."

I learned this in clinic as everything rushed to my head and I realized what had happened. I was looking at that 3-D-rendered scan on a computer screen, and as I rotated the skull image up, down, and all around, I saw those two rubber bands as clear as day, and my heart nearly dropped out of my chest onto the floor beneath me.

In the clinic room next door was Cheyenne, whose CT was pulled up in front of me and who had, by that point, happily reached eleven years of age. By her mom's account, prior to her emergency surgery she had always been a carefree spirited child who loved to dance "like no one was watching." Until her presentation months before, she had been a typical and healthy active redhead with a happy if not slightly sarcastic disposition.

I had first met Cheyenne on the pediatric ward at our children's hospital as she flailed around in her bed. Her fever was around 102, she was unresponsive, and she had just finished up a grand mal seizure a few seconds before I walked in. Her eyes were closed. Her breaths were long and noisy, rasping, as if she were stuck on the exhalation phase only. Cheyenne's mom was pacing the side of the bed. She looked to be in her early thirties, her hair graying around the edges and it appeared as if she had been up for days and worrying even longer than that.

"What are you going to do?" she asked me the moment I introduced myself.

Before I could answer, she asked me again, more forcefully, "What are you going to do?"

The ward nurse, with several other patients to care for, was coming in and out of the room, trying to work as many tasks as possible. She placed oxygen on Cheyenne's nose, and in her confused state Cheyenne would immediately yank the nasal cannula off of her face. The nurse connected anti-seizure meds into her IV that the primary team had recently ordered. She also turned to ask me what we wanted to do. The primary team was on their way, she said.

My current resident had been called because a CT scan done as a workup by the ward team for Cheyenne's worsening overnight fevers and mental status changes had just shown an infection along the surface of her brain under some pressure, known as a subdural empyema. He felt she needed to go to the OR emergently. He was 100 percent correct.

I had been in a meeting, one of many that day that were back to back, and stepped out when the seriousness of the call was clear.

"Call the OR," I said to him. "We need to go now."

To the nurse: "Call the ICU team, please. She's going to need to be intubated fairly soon."

To Mom: "Let's step outside for just a moment. The nurse and my resident will stay here next to her." I looked up to see her oxygen saturations hovering around 92 percent, the pulsing tone of the sat monitor lower than normal.

The nurse had wisely already called the ICU team, and the fellow, resident, respiratory tech, ICU nurse, and medical student came rushing up the stairs and spilled out into the hall, quickly orienting themselves to the right room. They saw me and came down the hall rolling more monitors and carrying various medicines arranged in medical versions of tackle boxes.

"We're taking her to the OR soon," I told them.

The neurosurgery resident popped his head out of the room and said, "OR is on the way."

I looked back at Cheyenne's mother, who was terrified but somehow relieved.

"I've been saying she's sick, Doctor. For days. Just getting worse and worse." It was spilling out of her now. "Headaches and acting out. Now this spell she's had. Is she going to make it?"

"She has something called a subdural empyema," I said back, quickly. "It's an infection along the surface of her brain collected up on the top, just off to the left side. She is very sick. We need to go in and drain it."

"How?"

"We have to remove a square area of bone, open up the covering of the brain, take some cultures to find out what this is, and then carefully irrigate out the infected fluid to get the pressure off. Then the antibiotics have to do their job."

"You are going now?"

"Yes, ma'am. We are going now."

She paused briefly, letting the enormousness of the moment wash over her.

"Good," she said matter-of-factly. "Take care of my baby."

In the OR, I made an incision that stayed behind her hairline all the way across the top of her head. In order to expose enough skull to do the craniotomy, I placed a rolled-up sponge under the outside of the base of the skin flap like all the times before, then temporarily sutured medium-sized sterile rubber bands into the inside of the flap and looped them around a metal bar secured to the sides of the bed and arching up and over our patient. Easy. Quick. We were at the drilling stage in five minutes.

The infection was worse than I'd expected from the CT. When we opened up the dura, pus came spilling out up and over the surgical field and down the drapes onto the floor. A medical student observing the anesthesia team for the week had looked up over the drapes at the wrong time and had to sit down and put his head between his legs to keep from passing out. Once we had suctioned most of the pus away, the brain beneath was angry, red, and irritated, and the tiny blood vessels running up and down the crevices of the brain were dilated in the same way the vessels appear in an irritated red eye. Tiny bits of infection stuck to the surface of the brain and the pia. Any attempt to suction or gently irrigate them away resulted in bleeding from the dilated and friable vessels. If it had been us playing the children's game Operation, all the little buzzers would have been going off, and the lightbulb nose would have exploded.

On top of all that, within a minute of the dura being opened, the brain very slowly began to swell.

"Lower the pCO_2," we called out, signaling for anesthesia to increase the respiratory rate and blow off more carbon dioxide in an attempt to stop the swelling. "Raise the head of the bed." These maneuvers can reduce brain swelling just enough to buy you time to get your job done and get out.

We harvested a nearby piece of pericranium and quickly sewed it into place with a few interrupted sutures to give the brain room to expand. We placed a small plastic tube to act as a drain down into the space alongside the brain where much of the infection had been. I decided to leave the bone flap out because we wanted to have space for the brain to swell out a bit to keep the pressure inside the skull from going too high. With the pCO_2 change, the head elevation, and the patch, things looked fine. Closure would be a matter of sewing up the skin on the inner and outer edges. All was stable. I began to think I could make the end of a meeting that I had scheduled for this hour. What in the world it was about I cannot even recall.

"You comfortable?" I asked my resident. "Okay to close up the rest of the skin?"

"Yes, sir," he replied, busying himself with irrigating out any remaining bone dust from the original craniotomy.

I walked out of the OR, confident that we had done what we had intended to do. I updated the mom, who by that point had been joined by family.

"Things will be tough for the next week," I said. "She will swell for a couple of days, and we will need to keep her on the breathing tube." I told her that we placed a tiny wire monitor in her brain to keep an eye on the pressure and be able to treat it with medication if needed.

The next three days were as rocky as anticipated. Her brain pressure went up and down. The antibiotics gradually took control of the infection, though, and within a few days her breathing tube was removed, and by the next week she was speaking in sentences and slowly asking for her favorite food.

It would only be after weeks of antibiotics and a few months of recovery that I was ready to put a 3-D-printed implant into the craniotomy defect. I felt that with the amount of infection present before, her native bone flap would be unlikely to heal without a problem, so I elected to get a special thin-cut CT so that a plastic composite piece could be 3-D printed, sterilized, and used to replace her bone. It was on that scan that I saw what had been left inside.

Somehow, we had failed to remove the two rubber bands during the closure, and somehow there was no hint of them on any prior imaging, and somehow, thankfully, she had cleared her infection even with the foreign bodies present.

I couldn't believe what I saw. I was in the middle of my busy clinic staring at a computer screen showing my mistake with nurses and students coming in and out of the room around me and each exam room full and me already running my typical one hour behind.

Are you kidding me? I thought to myself.

I called the head of our neuro OR team. No, I was told, the rubber bands are not counted before closure. That is not the protocol.

I had no choice but to tell the mother, straight up, there in clinic. We'd have to go in again and get them out. Thank heavens, we could do it at the same time we placed the skull implant and it wouldn't necessitate an extra procedure.

I walked into the exam room. There sat Cheyenne next to her mother. She was dressed up, a beret over the shorter red hair where we had clipped it months ago. There was an indentation underneath, where the bone was absent and the pressure now normal. They both stood up and smiled.

I was briefly shocked into forgetting my news. I had last seen her right before she was discharged home with close outpatient physical therapy. At that point she was slowly reaching out for a coloring marker and being spoon-fed apple sauce. She was still weak on the left side and only just starting to reach out with that hand. Most of us had recommended a stay in an inpatient rehabilitation unit out of state, but her mom said, "She isn't going to need as much help as y'all think. You don't know how strong-willed my Cheyenne is."

It was clear to me at that moment that her mother had been exactly right. What I saw when I walked in that clinic room was a remarkably healthy-looking teenager (with a slightly wonky haircut of my own making) smiling and thanking me. Her mom, standing next to her, beamed. Before I could respond, she moved us together for a photo.

I have to tell her.

"Say, 'CHEESE!'"

I have to tell her.

"A great picture," she said. "This is the doctor who saved your life, Cheyenne," her mom said, tearing up.

I wanted to stay right in that moment just a little longer. I could decide to not tell her, just clipping out the two rubber bands on the way in for the next procedure. None would be the wiser.

I let the excitement quiet down for a moment.

"There is something that I do need to tell you," I said.

When I had finished with the news, Cheyenne's mom sat down in the chair with her head down. This time, I noticed she was dressed entirely different from the times I had seen her in the hospital. Today, she wore a cardigan sweater and had slightly longer hair pulled back with a hair clasp that was lacquered, black on the outside and burnt orange showing on the edges. My mind filled the subsequent silence with thoughts that it looked like something my father would have brought back to my mother on one of his flights to Japan along with that heavy clay cooking oven and the beautiful spherical glass fishing buoy that sits next to the back door of the home I grew up in.

Before I had realized it, she looked up. Her face was brighter. She stood up and pulled her daughter in close. A tear rolled down her face.

"You saved my baby," she said. "My baby is here because of what you did that day."

"But I should have . . . ," I started to say.

She cut in. "I don't care if you left your car keys up there, Dr. Wellons. Look at her."

Cheyenne put her hand up to her head in mock astonishment: "I don't feel any car keys up there." She smiled and shook her head. "Wouldn't they jingle around when I turned my head?"

AFTER THE LAST surgery, during which we used those same rubber bands left there to retract the skin again, dissected out the bone defect without getting into the underlying brain (due, I like to think, to that patch we had placed in haste on our way out last time), fit the implant perfectly into the skull defect, and clipped out the two rubber bands when done, the scrub nurse and circulator counted the rubber bands in addition to the needles and sponges as part of the new protocol.

"We have two additional rubber bands in the count," they proudly announced when done.

Cheyenne stayed a single night in the hospital and went home the next day. I followed her for a while in clinic over the next year, gradually spacing out the visits with each great-looking follow-up CT scan. After the fourth such visit, it was time to release her from clinic. She no longer needed to see me on a routine basis.

This is an important time for the patient, the parent, and the surgeon. Both the patient and the parent can draw a line in the sand and say, I am done with this chapter of my life. For the surgeon, it marks the end of the time when you get to witness someone you've helped come back, then move forward. Those are the meaningful relationships. You come to miss hearing about school and what book they are reading. You miss seeing them grow up and hearing about their life now able to be lived because you did what you were trained to do. But of course, that is just as it is supposed to be. Somehow all the goodness and grace now interwoven over the years travels back to the past. The past where the earliest version of your story together is playing out, with all the unfolding intensity and urgency that emergency pediatric neurosurgery can have. And I recognize that this next part may not be typical pediatric neurosurgeon thinking (but I suspect that it is). That goodness and grace somehow reveal themselves to me right in that moment when I know the child must have the surgery to survive and that it is up to me to do it. I can see just the haziest version of a life to be lived, the relief in the parents' eyes during recovery, the joy of the later years now re-attained, and finally the discharge from clinic into the rest of life. I cannot explain it any better than that. I know it sounds nonsensical, the future influencing the past. But in my own mind that cycle exists, pushing me forward into the otherwise unknown.

At the end of her very last appointment, it was Cheyenne who stood up one last time to thank me. She reached out with her hands—those hands that had been flailing about wildly that first day in her hospital bed. She swept both of my hands into hers, holding them both out in front of us. Right then, as if said anew, I heard her mom's words in the clinic those many months ago granting me permission to forgive myself and move on.

You saved my baby.

It is for this reason that when I see a simple rubber band, like the one I keep on my desk at work next to the photo of Cheyenne and me that her mother took those many years ago, I am reminded of the immense and time-transcending power of giving and receiving, of love and grace and forgiveness, and the way that all of them bind us together on this earth.

9

Last Place

IT WAS AROUND 5:45 in the morning as I topped a long hill on the interstate. One of my favorite things to do in the early years of my career was to get done with a busy workweek at the hospital and at the last minute find a short "sprint" triathlon somewhere nearby on a Saturday morning. Then that Friday night after dinner, I would pack up my gear, stick my bike on top of my Subaru, and prepare to head out the next morning, sometimes leaving as early as 3:00 A.M. to get to various places in time to register and set up my transition area for the race. It was a great way to get out of the confines of the hospital and decompress.

Typically, I was happy to finish in the top half overall of those races. As a kid, I was never particularly great at any one sport, but did pride myself on the ability to do many different types of sports. I could ski, surf, fence, and beat my older cousin Brad at table tennis. I suppose that is why I enjoyed triathlons. Three sports combined into one. Great exercise for the sake of exercise. That day, however, was different, because I was eager to finish high up in my age-group. I had actually pre-registered and been training hard and wanted to put up my best race times. As I drove, my thoughts drifted to getting in and out of both transitions quickly.

I remember the sun rising behind me on the near-empty inter-state as I headed due west. I saw a cloud of dust on the median as

I came over the crest of the hill. Then I saw that same cloud of dust leap into the air, twisting to throw out a woman at the apex of its heave, and land crashing to the ground. As the dust and smoke cleared, there was left a crumpled minivan on its side, its undercarriage facing me.

It took a few seconds for me to realize that I had just seen an accident. I wrenched the car over to the fire lane, opened my car door, and ran to the van. There were bits and pieces of these people's lives strewn about the road and median: a cracked DVD player—the kind that fits over the back of a car's seat—a worn dinosaur doll, a pink pillow now half-soaked in a spreading pool of filmy brown liquid, a package of unopened lunch meat. I ran past all of it.

Cars coming from the other direction had started to slow and pull over. Half a dozen people now ran across the wide median, still at least thirty seconds away, as they made their way through the grass, trees, and intervening drainage ditch.

I arrived well before the others. A man lay across the front seat, his right ear just hanging on by the earlobe. Bright red blood gushed down the side of his face in waves from an open neck wound. Someone helped me get him out of the car and lay him on the grass a few yards away. I don't remember how we got him out. I do remember the warmth of the blood across the side of my face. I held pressure against the side of his neck, where I assumed he was bleeding out from a tear in his carotid artery. The others brought two more and laid them next to us. I straddled the man and pressed hard. He called out in pain. Soon only venous blood oozed around my fingers. He was breathing and his eyes were moving in all directions under his closed lids.

I looked up to see a long-haired blond toddler scratched about the face but awake and crying as she leaned into a middle-aged woman's embrace.

"She okay?" I yelled up to her as she stood over me.

"Found her in a car seat," she yelled back to me and rocked the child in her arms.

I reached up instinctively to feel the child's neck for a step-off in the alignment that would have signified a spine fracture. She was moving and awake; my exam would be mostly meaningless. I reached up and felt no issues, leaving what appeared to be a giant bloody handprint on the back of her neck.

"I got this," the woman said. "You take care of them." She walked away from the scene a few feet and faced into the sun. She was wearing scrubs and a name tag, so I figured she was a healthcare worker of some type, heading to or from work this morning at a local hospital.

I looked over to a man wearing a checkered short-sleeve shirt.

"*You*," I yelled. "I need you to hold pressure here," and I put his hand over the man's neck. "This much," showing him how much with my own hand. "And keep his neck straight, no matter what."

To the woman with him, I said, "I need you to hold his leg as straight as you can and hold pressure here." As I said it, I reduced his knee that had been at an unnatural ninety-degree angle, off to one side. The patient yelled out briefly, but was silent again. "Talk to him if he wakes up. Calm him down," I said.

The person on the ground just next to the man was a teenage girl who was fighting against two people who had her pinned down, trying to keep her still. She was screaming and crying.

I got down right in her face. "*Let me check you*," I yelled. Her color was good, she was moving everything, and she was clearly breathing. Her neck felt fine. No pain there that she related to me.

"Let her up," I said. "She will hurt herself worse fighting."

They released her and she sat forward, crying.

"*You*," I said to a twentysomething man in a tie-dyed T-shirt, "just stay with her. Talk to her."

The final person in the row was a different story. I assumed she

was the wife and mother. She was the one ejected from the vehicle as it rolled. Her skin and lips were a deepening shade of blue,
and she was taking short shallow breaths, more like gulps of air.
This is more than bleeding from a wound that I need to hold pressure on, I
thought. How different this was from the OR, where airway, breathing, and bleeding control are expected. No anesthesiologist or nurse
anesthetist. No circulating nurse or scrub techs to hand me sterile
and near-perfect task-specific instruments while we work the day
away, sometimes serious under the microscope and sometimes closing up and listening to music. This wasn't even like the chaos of
the emergency department, where the patients often arrive already
intubated and we come down to whisk them away to the CT scanner or the operating room.

"WHY AREN'T YOU HELPING HER?" The teenager's nearby
scream broke my train of thought.

I put my ear to her chest and heard nothing on the right. Most
likely, she had a tension pneumo- or hemothorax. Either the lung
had been injured and air was leaking out into the space between her
lungs and her chest wall, or one of the large vessels in the chest had
been severed, and the lung was being pushed over by a massive clot
of blood. Puncturing her chest wall with a needle or instrument of
some kind would release the pressure on her lungs and heart and
save her at least temporarily. If it was a pneumothorax, then releas-
ing the trapped air would restore respiration and circulation of oxygenated blood. If it was trapped blood from a torn great vessel, she
would die quickly from blood loss. The standard approach was to
try to decompress, because the right guess would save the patient
and the wrong one would kill a patient unlikely to survive such a
terrific injury anyway.

The issue at hand was that in my sweatshirt and pants and with
no medical kit whatsoever, I had nothing to decompress her with. I
have trauma surgeon friends who carry a large-gauge IV needle in
their car to use in just this situation. I remembered my folding Allen

wrench set under the seat of my triathlon bike that was mounted on top of my car. I sent someone for it, thinking that I would soon need to puncture her chest wall about a hand's breadth below the underarm. Where do the trauma folks put the chest tube, again? It had been more than ten years since my intern year in the true trenches. *This*, I thought, *is not going to go well.*

That's when I heard the distant wail of the approaching ambulances. Let me be very clear here. That far-off siren of an approaching ambulance that you know is coming to you, to help, is a sweet sound when you are in the field. Particularly when you are in the field in sweatpants, with only a multipurpose bike tool and two rapidly dying people. The mother's heart rate was fast. I was having a hard time multiplying the number of pulse beats in ten seconds times six. I was drenched in sweat. My glasses were steamed up, but I could at least see that most of her bleeding from her abrasions, or road rash, was minimal. But there was no doubt that she would die soon if we did not get her chest decompressed.

As soon as the ambulances pulled up, I got up and jogged down the row of our patients, each now being tended to by two or three people. Everything still seemed so chaotic. The woman holding the toddler was nearby and calmly walking toward the ambulances.

I yelled out to the first paramedic I saw, "I'm a surgeon. Middle-aged woman, ejected from car, with rapid shallow respirations. No breath sounds on the right. I believe she has a tension pneumothorax and needs a decompression or a stat chest tube. She is the sickest."

The first medic leaned down to listen to her chest with a stethoscope. He then motioned to a second one who had just emerged from the back of the ambulance with a gurney.

"Tension pneumo," he yelled. "On the right. Lips blue. Get her in the truck and get her chest decompressed now. Then intubate her."

He looked back to me.

"Middle-aged man," I said. "Deep laceration to neck, maybe to the carotid. We are holding pressure. At least a liter of blood loss that I could see. Ear avulsed. Right leg tib fib ninety-degree angulated fracture, in line, no traction. I do not know about the pulses.

"Teenage girl," I continued. "Scratched up and bruised, but we couldn't keep her still. She is walking around the scene." I pointed to the tie-dye-wearing twentysomething who was still with her, walking next to her, doing his best to comfort her.

The head paramedic sent off two more teams with gurneys and looked at me, his right eyebrow arching. We could hear the far-off sound of the approaching medevac helicopter.

"One more," I said. "A female toddler. Found in her car seat. I did feel her neck. She was moving everything a little while ago." I pointed toward the woman with the child who was just handing her off to a paramedic near the ambulance.

"It all just happens so fast. So damn fast. How in the world do you guys do this?" I asked him.

The lead paramedic paused before answering, smiling just for a split second, then said to me loudly over the helicopter making its landing approach nearby, "Doc, you want to fly the chopper, too?"

The woman's lung was quickly decompressed in the ambulance, and she was taken by air from the scene directly to the nearest Level I trauma center. The father was taken in another helicopter with a large clean pressure dressing on the side of his neck and head being held in place by a paramedic. The children were loaded up in the ground ambulances, placed on backboards and stretchers with cervical spine collars in place, and taken to the nearest hospital for quick assessment per protocol before being transferred to a children's hospital forty-five minutes away.

As the ambulances and emergency trucks began to make their way down the fire lanes back to their local home bases, I looked up to see long lines of backed-up traffic in both directions. Some of them heading west had bikes on top of the cars. I realized that many of these making their way past me were headed to my race.

I walked up to the road toward my car and saw two racers driving in their triathlon outfits, bikes racked in the back of their truck, slowly making their way in a single file down the road. They stared at me and rolled down the window a little hesitantly. I realized right then that I was covered in blood: my hands, arms, shirt, and all down the front of my pants.

"Looks like you've had a busy day," the driver said.

"I think I'm going to be late for the race," I said, wiping my hands on my sweatpants.

"We called the organizer when the traffic started backing up," the passenger leaned over and said. "They know about the wreck. They said they are going to postpone the start forty-five minutes."

"When you get there, just ask them to hold it fifteen minutes more," I said. "Just fifteen minutes more."

I did get to the race start, and they had indeed held the starting gun for me to arrive. I ran my bike into the transition area, shed my bloody clothes, upended my race bag, and scraped everything into a pile in my assigned area. There was a smattering of applause from the racers who had lined up for the time trial start. I picked out my goggles and swim cap and ran to the race start. I did not check my tire pressure. Nor did I put my gel in my left shoe or my sunglasses in my bike helmet. I still started well enough in the water, holding my own and passing a few as I came around the final buoy. During the bike loop, I began to fade, every bit of adrenaline within me depleted. In fact, I couldn't even find my assigned spot in the transition area and wasted almost an entire minute looking for it. People who were initially clapping for me started guiding me as I ran up and down the aisles trying to find my running shoes and gear amid hundreds of similar-looking piles.

During the entire race, I kept thinking how different things were in the field. How raw and chaotic and bloody and human. Screaming and spittle and gravel and grass blades, all merged together. Split-second decisions in the field were the rule, not the exception like in the operating room. *My gosh,* I thought, *I take out brain tumors in kids. Why am I so affected here?* I felt so changed in how I thought about trauma. *How can I pass judgment on a first responder ever again for not keeping the neck in line, or not splinting the leg once reduced, or missing an acute abdomen when they are in the middle of the chaos of it all? I never even did a freaking full neurologic exam, only bits and pieces here and there.* Waves of thought and doubt from the early morning washed over me. *Did I do the right things? Did the whole family make it?* I wanted as much of the happy ending as possible.

I proceeded to drink too much water at the start of the run and cramped, and then, at the turnaround of the three-mile out and back, I sprained my ankle. I sat on the trail and taped it with duct tape someone had at the water station. I resumed a lurching jog and crossed the finish line last. Completely last. I don't even remember an actual time recorded. I think they might have even taken some of the timing mats up. It was by far my worst finish for that race distance ever.

Well after the award ceremony was over and the post-race food was eaten, I finished gathering up my gear strewn about the transition zone and slowly limped to my car holding on to my bike stem. The race organizers were rolling up the temporary orange plastic fences and the finish line flags in the background. Many of the early finishers had already pulled out of the parking lot. A nearby paramedic crew was loading up their truck with their unused medical equipment. Race protocol dictates that there is always at least one ambulance or fireman medic team assigned per race in case someone is injured along the route or a racer starts having heart problems from pushing themselves too hard. I walked over to where they were packing up. I caught a quick glimpse of an empty and clean gurney being loaded into the ambulance.

"Did you hear anything about a car accident on the interstate early this morning?" I asked the nearest paramedic.

"Yep," he nodded. "Family of four. They all made it. Every one of them."

I heard, then felt, a rush of blood in my ears. I leaned up against my bike for the few seconds it took to clear. The sun was now nearly directly above the lake, the heat of the day upon us.

"Good race today?" he asked, closing the back doors of the ambulance.

"Yes. It was great," I answered, smiling and turning back to my car. "I came in last place."

———◆———

10

See One, Do One, Teach One

I T IS THE fall of 2016 and I am in Brisbane, Australia, in an operating room standing off to the side of the sterile field with my surgical loupes and headlight on, waiting to operate on a fetus inside the womb, the first time this remarkable but risky procedure is to be performed in this part of the world. I am there with Martin Wood, my Australian pediatric neurosurgeon counterpart, whom I met thirty-six hours before. Both of us have our arms crossed. Martin is watching the monitor showing the ongoing exposure of the glistening surface of the uterus, and I am staring down at the floor thinking through the surgical steps to come, steeling myself for our part of the operation.

This is the most difficult moment in any operation, in my opinion, that final wait, when you have gone over each part of the procedure repeatedly, and there is nothing else left to do but begin. When you are laser focused and ready like this, that anxiety peaks, as if you were hovering over a precipice having wrangled up all your courage to jump out into the abyss. But there you wait. The moment you finally start, it just . . . dissipates. You concentrate on one step, then the next, all the while managing any unexpected issue presenting itself. All of this is of course heightened today because of the whole first-in-the-country issue. But today, like any other, our signal will be the firing of the surgical stapler, when the maternal-fetal surgeons open the wall of the uterus to expose the fetus, then rotate the exposed spinal cord into view.

There are many more people in the OR than I am used to. To be honest, I have never liked having people watch me operate. I feel critiqued, as if they felt they could do it better, surgical training or not. I recognize the ridiculousness of this when I am later finished in the OR and thinking over how all went well, or some unexpected issue was managed appropriately. I feel as if I were the only surgeon in the world who would prefer to operate in a closet with the smallest team possible, then celebrate with the family when everything was done and walk away quietly. As time has gone by in my career, that is less and less possible.

Today two teams from opposite sides of the world have come together to perform the operation, intrauterine surgery for a myelomeningocele closure, or in less medical terms, surgery on a still-developing fetus while in the womb to repair the exposed maldeveloped spinal cord, the hallmark of spina bifida. There is a mix of anxiety and excitement pervasive among everyone present. More than a hundred people were involved in making this happen, from those who raised the money to bring us over to the sizable OR team available that day, and of course the brave Australian couple who had agreed to take the risk. The procedure was taking place on a Sunday, a less busy day in the ORs, to allow personnel to focus on this one event. Several adjacent ORs were set up with closed-circuit video and rows of chairs full of hospital employees, doctors, nurses, support staff, anyone who wanted to be present for the perceived Australian medical history being made.

Suddenly the crack of the surgical stapler being fired sounds out as the uterine wall opening is extended.

I turn to Martin and nod. Silently, we both head to the scrub sink to wash our hands.

I am here because our Vanderbilt Fetal Center surgery team was asked to help a newly commissioned group in Brisbane perform that part of the world's first intrauterine operation for spina bifida repair. Spina bifida is an age-old metabolic issue concerning folic acid production occurring in a subset of pregnant women that affects the developing spinal cord of the fetus. It is the reason that years ago folate was added to bread. If there is not enough folic acid around in the early stages of pregnancy, even including the brief time before women can know they are pregnant, the spinal canal does not completely close at the lower end during development. The affected spinal canal remains open and exposed to the outside. In addition, none of the nerves work in the areas affected. The legs and muscles form, even the normal-appearing nerves, but without a functioning spinal cord, it does not matter. Until fetal surgery was found to be effective, spina bifida was treated in the first few days after delivery with surgery on the infant's exposed spinal cord to separate it from the surrounding skin and then close the layers of muscle, fat, and skin over the top. Most of the children would then go on to develop hydrocephalus. They also have difficulty walking, if they can at all, lack bladder or bowel continence, develop prominent and debilitating spinal deformities requiring corrective surgery, and have a host of other developmental issues. It was only in the mid-twentieth century that medical science advanced to the point that these children would be able to grow into adulthood and not die along the way mainly from hydrocephalus or renal failure.

It is important here to delve further into the role that hydrocephalus and shunt placement play in these patients. A shunt is basically a small tube with a pressure- or volume-regulated valve placed under the skin that diverts the backed-up CSF from the enlarged ventricles of the brain to empty in the abdomen, where it is ultimately absorbed back into the body. When they work they are terrific, but as parents and pediatric neurosurgeons (and ER doctors) know, they can be finicky. Sometimes that finickiness leads to a slowly building headache, culminating in a visit to the local emergency department and operating room, and sometimes, thankfully rarely, it leads to the child suffering acute shunt failure in the night and never waking up again. This constant awareness of suffering and catastrophe in addition to negative health effects from the lack of mobility leads to a lower life expectancy over time.

As the new millennium approached, a handful of surgeons and fetal specialists began to consider that there was more to be done to help these children, and that perhaps something could be done *even earlier than birth* to improve outcome. Animal studies and actual early human fetal interventions were being done by two main centers: the Children's Hospital of Philadelphia (CHOP) and Vanderbilt University. Both centers, working separately, had developed the idea of attempting to repair the spinal cord earlier than birth, *inside* the uterus, while critical development was still occurring. It had been shown that the intrauterine environment was toxic to the exposed spinal cord, because meconium and other fetal waste products could build up and cause scarring and neural damage that was thought to further worsen functional outcome. In addition, stopping the leakage of spinal fluid from around the defect appeared to reduce the development of hydrocephalus. While it may be impossible (for now) to intervene when the initial malformation occurs in those earliest weeks of pregnancy, perhaps stopping the exposure damage, as well as reducing the loss of spinal fluid into the amniotic fluid, would result in functional improvement.

The early results were promising. However, the main drawback was the risk of preterm birth, of delivery of the fetus prior to full term. This increases the risk across multiple organ systems, including the newborn lungs, gastrointestinal system, brain, and a host of other issues. At what point would the risk of preterm delivery outweigh the benefit of surgery on the developing fetus? Just on the brink of multiple centers for fetal surgery opening across North America, in the absence of clear data that the benefits outweighed the risks, the National Institutes of Health (NIH) stepped in. A moratorium would be placed on any new centers performing the operation. Only the original two, CHOP and Vanderbilt, and one additional center, the University of California, San Francisco, would be allowed to do the surgery, and this would be in the confines of a well-designed study. In addition, both fetal surgery and postnatal surgery—the traditional timing of surgery after delivery—would be performed, and strict guidelines would be followed for who was to be enrolled, the randomization process, how the surgery would be performed, and what the outcomes of interest would be. Then, over time, the results would be tallied and shared.

Vanderbilt's pediatric neurosurgeon Noel Tulipan, a quiet man, unassuming but relentless, had been a part of the two-person team at Vanderbilt working toward a feasible procedure in the early years. He, along with Joseph Bruner, a maternal-fetal medicine specialist, had done a great deal of work with the preclinical studies and were involved in every procedure done at Vanderbilt. Similar teams were standardized at the other two centers, as well as the surgical procedure itself, so as to ensure uniformity. Years went by as the trial unfolded. Many parents wanted fetal surgery, but without clear data the only way to be eligible was to enroll as a candidate in the trial, called MOMS—the Management of Myelomeningocele Study—and be randomized to either fetal or postnatal surgery, the chance of either equal for each patient.

MOMS was done well before I arrived at Vanderbilt. The study actually had to be halted, not because of complications of the procedure, but because the benefit of fetal surgery was deemed to be so great. As enrollment entered the final phases, enough results were in that it was clear it would be unethical to continue. All eligible mother-fetus dyads should have access to fetal surgery and no longer be under randomization to a possible postnatal closure. After the results of MOMS were published in *The New England Journal of Medicine,* to great fanfare, it became time to lift the moratorium on other centers performing the procedure. Dozens of teams from North America traveled to Vanderbilt and the other two centers to learn from the fetal teams. It was in this environment at Vanderbilt that I became involved. I was recruited to build up the Division of Pediatric Neurosurgery. Part of that was for me, over time, to assume Noel's role in the fetal surgery program as he was nearing retirement. It seemed like an interesting new world to explore, to add to my surgical repertoire. I was not aware at the time that Noel had been diagnosed with recurrent cancer and was undergoing experimental treatment and that his time unfortunately was limited.

The first case that I took part in, I scrubbed in to assist Noel. This is typical for the standard surgeon's progression: *See one, do one, teach one.* Even though I had done hundreds of postnatal closures before, operating on a fetus was like nothing I had ever experienced. The team at Vanderbilt, led by the maternal-fetal surgeon Kelly Bennett, was a close group, and I was not a part of them yet. They were wary of me, that was obvious. Noel, by this point in his career, had done the most fetal operations for spina bifida of anyone; I used to joke with him and say *more than anyone in the known galaxy.* I was clearly not him. Folding myself in would take time.

Then, soon after, there was another case with Noel. *Do one.* This time he assisted me. The tissue was entirely different at twenty-three weeks of gestation, akin to sewing wet tissue paper. The slightest wrong move would tear the fragile skin. I found myself calling out while operating, "Like this, Noel?" Or, "What do you think about this stitch, Noel?" I think the sheer magnitude of what I was involved in caused me to revert, just the littlest bit, to an earlier version of my surgical self, less confident, more in need of validation. Just like the one before, all went well.

Then a next case soon afterward where the resident scrubbed to assist me while Noel watched—*teach one*—and suddenly Noel was done. At his retirement party a little while later, he was feted for a career pushing fetal surgery forward, his résumé a testament to his willing it into being. Partners, nurses, and colleagues from all over the medical center attended to pay their respects to his surgical prowess and innovative career. Then, a few months later, Noel was dead. One year shy of sixty-five. He was buried in a quiet family ceremony, and the team grieved his loss. He had kept his illness a secret until the end. I was left to pick up where he had left off. He, having done more of these procedures than anyone in the world. I, by that point, had done a handful.

Months later, I had gained the confidence of the team. We had published some key papers together in the field of fetal surgery, and over time they began to trust my judgment and surgical ability in the operating room. I felt as though we were picking up well where things had been left off. Teams still came to visit, including many of the pediatric neurosurgeons I knew, to watch and learn the technique. Noel over time had evolved the actual surgical steps into a more streamlined version than in the MOMS trial, and it shaved time off the closure part itself. I no longer felt under the same degree of scrutiny. Most pediatric neurosurgeons came with the skill set of repairing myelomeningoceles after birth and, once acclimated to the smaller size and more fragile tissue, gained technical ability quickly. The teams, which typically also included a maternal-fetal specialist as well as an anesthesiologist specializing in obstetrical anesthesia, mostly came to learn the uterine opening anyway. Opening an intact uterus in a pregnant patient is not standard teaching in an obstetrics residency training program. One of the earlier papers we had published showed a reduction in premature delivery with the techniques the Vanderbilt team leader, Kelly Bennett, had developed. Kelly herself had taken over from Joseph Bruner years before when he moved on to another institution. Our new team began to settle into a routine. Several groups from around the country and even the world came to visit us.

Then came the call from Australia. This time the group in Brisbane wanted our whole OR team, all seven of us, to come to them (they had visited months before) and merge our teams together in the operating room. This, obviously, was not a common request. In addition, the operation was scheduled three weeks away due to the team there just having been referred the patient that day, and all of us needed visas, and temporary medical licenses, to clear our own schedules at work, and several other tall orders that we only vaguely took into consideration at the time we agreed to do it. It took a full-court press to make all of this happen, but soon enough, and thanks to our administrative assistants, we were appropriately documented for a medical visit to Australia.

Our entourage consisted of myself and six others: Kelly Bennett, the lead maternal-fetal surgeon; Stephane Braun from the department of plastic surgery, who was present to assist with several stages of the procedure; and Ray Paschall from the department of anesthesiology, who was there to "pass the gas" (not so easy considering that a fetus is safely ensconced behind the placental barrier). Ray had been involved with the fetal spina bifida effort since before the days of MOMS and was one of two vestiges of that original team. The other, the pediatric cardiologist Ann Kavanaugh-McHugh, was along as well to monitor the fetal heart during the surgery itself via an echocardiogram performed in real time during the actual operation. This would allow us to be aware of early signs of fetal distress that can be seen by a trained eye and are important to the anesthesia and surgical teams in order to respond quickly to correct. The last two, Alicia Crum and Melissa Broyles, were not physicians but were critical to the effort nonetheless. Alicia does the vast majority of the fetal ultrasounds in the clinic, and specifically the echo of the fetal heart in the OR. She stands to my left, scrubbed, with a sterile ultrasound wand on the uterine wall, and we often either bump elbows or find our arms entwined as we do our jobs. Melissa, the scrub nurse who also works in general surgery and urology in the Vanderbilt main ORs, is the scrub who is most involved with these operations and passionate about her work. These two women are so valued that both have to be available in order for us to schedule a fetal case, at home or on the other side of the world.

I viewed myself as a bit of an impostor as we boarded the airplane for Hong Kong. I had not made my life's work the development of this field. I had come late to the party, yet here I was. Being a longtime fan of the early days of the space program, I unwittingly chose the movie *Apollo 13* to watch on the flight over. This led me of course to the unshakable feeling of being like Jack Swigert, the Apollo 13 astronaut who famously replaced Ken Mattingly prior to launch.

When we arrived in Hong Kong, our flight was delayed and we were rerouted through Sydney, and then on to Brisbane. The members of the Australian Health Practitioner Regulation Agency, the group specially convened for this historic moment tasked with granting our temporary Australian medical licenses, waited in their boardroom and by speakerphone for us to arrive. With luggage in tow and pushing thirty hours of travel, we were driven over to their headquarters. We had been told to bring either original or notarized copies of all of our degrees, licenses, and medical board memberships. One of the highlights of that meeting was seeing Ann, the seasoned pediatric cardiologist (and mother of four adult children), take out her original still-rolled-up diplomas and graduate school degrees and present them to the officials.

"Hey," she said as the official unrolled each one like a scroll with a surprised look on her face, holding each at arm's length like the town crier, "I'd rather have pictures of my family in my office than these stuffy things. We have a pile in the attic for these." This immediately made me reevaluate all the stuffy things on my own office walls there to impress no one but me.

Soon we were approved and sent on our way, but despite our exhausted state not quite yet to bed. We met our hosts, pairing up with our counterparts at a dinner that we learned was planned in our honor. After a coffee as my before-dinner drink, I sat across from Martin, the local pediatric neurosurgeon. He had a young family, like me, and a wife who was also a physician. We had been out of training for around the same time and found that we had a great deal in common. I listened as hard as I could, doing my best to stay awake. Martin was quite funny, and I took to him quickly. I tried to think of the old standby stories of growing up in Mississippi. I remember thinking, *But I am a fun guy, too,* as I fell asleep in my chair waiting for dessert.

The next day began at 8:00 A.M. with a simulation. There were more than thirty people in the OR, and together the two teams performed every aspect of the simulation, step by step. We passed on our collective knowledge and experience to the team over a four-hour period. They, in turn, informed us of the culture specific to Australian operating rooms. A few of the instruments had alternate names, and some of the nursing titles were different; the Australians call their circulating nurses "scouts." (Yes, I tried it out when I got back to the United States, and no, I did not try it again after the first time.) In retrospect, this simulation was critical, similar to a pilot training on a flight simulator, for both standard and emergency scenarios. When we felt we had it down after several run-throughs and even an unexpected staged placental abruption and delivery, we all felt as ready as we could be. We then progressed to a critical next step, meeting the prospective patient and her husband.

Unlike many families that we consult on in the States, it was only the two of them. No other family around the conference table to weigh in. They sat close together, she with a loose scarf on her head and clearly in the late second trimester of her pregnancy, visible even through her long colorful dress. Her husband held her hand and offered her water as we walked in. Both radiated confidence in their decisions up to this point that had put them in this place. I noticed there were no tissue boxes on the table—the time for tears and making hard choices had come and gone. They were both already highly informed of the data behind what we were proposing to do, felt comfortable and pleased with our final recommendation to proceed. The conversation took around thirty minutes. Once done, we were standing up to leave, and I saw the man turn to face his wife. They closed their eyes and held hands. The door closed behind us.

The next day began early for everyone. Start time was 7:00 A.M., which meant that the OR staff, anesthesia team, and patient were all getting started hours earlier. Martin and I had struck up a quick friendship in the thirty-six hours since our arrival. It was very important to both teams that the Americans not come in and just do the whole thing ourselves and go home. We hadn't traveled all this way for that. Rather, after we left, Martin and his team would have to be able to perform this surgery themselves and also likely teach other teams in this part of the world.

A great deal of information can be transferred through conversations around a cup of coffee or a whiteboard, simulations run, or observation of surgery during collegial visits, but I had never been a part of anything like this in which two teams were merged entirely for an operation, zipped up for the one procedure, to be unzipped afterward. To be clear, there was significant risk here. Risk to the unborn child—intrauterine closure of spina bifida is the only fetal procedure done for a nonlethal issue. Indeed, there are very few actual indications for fetal surgery at all. Other procedures for other fetal defects came and went, the risk outweighing the benefit each time. But thanks to the NIH, and all who participated in MOMS, here the risk of preterm birth was worth the future benefit to the child. Yet today failure would not only have an impact on this fetus, this mother. Failure would be catastrophic for every child in this part of the world who could potentially benefit from the procedure, as the inevitable fetal death or complication would lead to finger-pointing and greater scrutiny.

But today, each step of the operation, done together as paired teams just as we had practiced it, started smoothly enough. Melissa had arrived at 4:30 A.M. to set up the complex instrument trays with two of the local nurses and watched over the sterility of the back table with the same zeal that we were used to at home. Ray worked with his Australian anesthesiologist counterpart on the appropriate IV lines and in delivering his particular method of anesthetic induction and maintenance that kept the uterus relaxed just enough during surgery. As the uterus was gradually exposed, Alicia skillfully glided the sterile ultrasound probe over its pink dome, transmitting a healthy fetus and heart images to Ann, set up with line of sight in the corner. Kelly meticulously led Glenn, her local maternal-fetal colleague and Australian team leader, through the uterine opening, minimizing damage to the muscle and quickly sewing the placental membranes up to the inner wall when identified.

While Martin and I stood off to the side, the significance of the next few minutes began to settle in. For the mother, the father, their unborn fetus, for us, for Glenn's team, for all the children that could one day be affected by this surgery here on this side of the world. I had just begun the final layer of closure in my mind, when the crack of the stapler signaled that it was our time to begin.

The room was quiet as we entered after scrubbing, hands up, palms in, fingers extended. We both wore surgical loupes and portable headlights in order to magnify and illuminate the area that we were to operate on. Often as neurosurgeons we would use an operating microscope for those reasons, and these are indeed marvelous devices but are large and unwieldy and have no place today. As we approached the table after drying our hands and gowning, we could hear the rhythmic tones of the mother's heartbeat emanating from the monitor. The pink uterus was exposed and approximately the size of a basketball. The abdominal skin, once taut from the underlying uterus, was now bunched up under the uterus, the yellow fat showing around the white sterile operative cloths—called sponges—laid over the remainder of the open abdomen. I was briefly aware of the sheer number of people watching around us. I quickly blocked it out.

As we stepped up, I nodded and greeted the other surgeons around the table, trying for just a moment to release the tension, which was palpable. I looked down to see the exposed spinal cord, the size of three grains of rice put together, suspended on a bubble of thin translucent tissue containing the spinal fluid. Martin and I quickly began to separate the tiny spinal cord and nerve roots from the surrounding skin where it was abnormally attached. Once that was completed, we turned our attention to the skin itself. Gentle dissection under the normal skin on both sides of the defect typically allows us to bring the midline together and cover the neural tissue with normal skin. Here, however, the base of the lesion was too far apart to accomplish that. Alicia and I had secretly suspected as much from the ultrasound done the day before, but it is hard to tell until you see things with your own eyes. This confirmed another reason why we were here, the experience needed to close a wider than normal defect in the back of a twenty-four-week fetus with a blood volume less than a quarter of a can of soda. To accomplish this, we would have to make extra incisions on the flank of the fetus that would allow the midline tissue enough laxity to enable the fetal skin to stretch across the lesion, but not under significant tension or the repair would fall apart prior to delivery.

"Stephane," I said to the plastic surgeon on our team, "I need you up here."

Martin moved to the side just enough and Stephane slid in. We had done this together multiple times before. The three of us made our extra incisions in the fetal flank and worked quickly.

Kelly leaned in to gently remind us of the time-sensitive nature of the operation: "The clock is ticking, boys."

The space in which we work is around the size of a tablespoon. There is a moment when Ann's voice rings out: The heart is underfilling as the extra incisions cause a tiny bit more bleeding than typical. The cardiac output drops slightly as the heart rate rises, an early sign of fetal stress. The room freezes, teetering on an edge familiar to seven of us alone, but in our tablespoon we carry on. With time, this passes. The flaps are done. Stephane steps to the side, and Martin moves back to the position across from me. The skin across the midline on both sides is now loose and supple, more than adequate to complete the repair. We slide in a tiny graft of collagen material underneath the skin, which will be incorporated over time into the dura surrounding the now freed-up spinal cord. The scrub nurse starts to hand me the needle driver; I motion for Martin to take it. Systematically, he sews up the back, advancing the needle three millimeters at a time until he is at the other end of the repair site.

"Let the record show," I say as he carefully ties the knot. "The first fetal myelomeningocele closed on Australian soil was by an Australian surgeon." I hear muffled clapping and exhalations around us.

Kelly steps in and quietly wisecracks, "Okay, hotshots, someone has to get us home. Now step back and go get us some coffee ready."

Over the next few hours, our patient awoke and spoke to her husband. Gradually, we allowed ourselves to feel the enormity of what we had done. That feeling after a successful complex surgery outstrips nearly every other intense emotion. It is a strong mix of relief and wonder that I often feel in the family consultation room outside the OR when sharing the results to relieved parents, or in the still, quiet space of the changing room late in the day. Here, on the other side of the world, with people we had not known until only a few days before, and the setting in which this was done (and in the haze of a completely destroyed sleep schedule), the feeling was remarkable.

We attended an excellent professional Australian Rules football game later that day, the rules of which I could never get straight, then had a relaxed dinner. The next morning, after a stable night, a press conference was called at which all of the major news networks appeared. Many focused on it being the first such operation in Australia, and then on the risk. I was tired; all of us were. Even the Australians had felt the weight of what those last days had brought. At the lectern, when asked about the risk of the procedure, I misspoke. Instead of saying what I had intended to say, that the procedure was just at "the edge of risk," I said "the edge of death." The quotation headlined the Australian news websites within the hour (much to my U.S. partners' delight and my chagrin). But as the story grew over the hours and days afterward, and the journalists realized what they truly had in this narrative, it became less about the sensational and more focused on where it should be, on the patients, on the teams working together, and on children with spina bifida and what can be done to lessen their burden.

Each fetal case is remarkable. Seeing life developing inside the womb, just a glimpse through this surgical window, is astounding on its own. But then being at a time when we can intervene in a way that makes a difference, and then *close that window* for a bit longer, that is a position that few people are allowed to be in, and I am awed by it. Each time I stand over the table putting the final stitches in, I am washed over by a sense of wonder. Wonder that this can be done and that, somehow, I have found my way to being a part of it. There are others better at this than me, certainly. As a surgeon, you learn that there is always someone a little better, a little faster, a little more adept at self-promotion. Indeed, as we have taught more and more centers the procedure, our own case count has dropped. But that was the deal at the very beginning of MOMS. Each center would stop except for three. Then, if MOMS showed success— which it certainly did—other centers would be eligible to learn and to start their own programs. What is the minimum number of fetal spina bifida operations a center needs to do each year? How to expand eligibility for the procedure? How to improve upon the procedure itself? These are all questions I am asked at the podium at national meetings as part of an "expert panel" or one-on-one by my colleagues. I cannot answer these alone. I can't do any of this alone. I prefer to focus on the wonder, and let this next generation of surgeons take up the arguments, find those answers, and push the field forward. I am content with my role in this journey. *See one, do one, teach one.*

11

Conversations

M OST CONVERSATIONS THAT pediatric neurosurgeons have
with parents when meeting them for the first time are usually the hardest things that parents have ever had to hear about their
children. *But he's always been healthy . . . She's never been sick a day of
her life . . . How is this happening?* Nowhere is that as true as in the
ED or in the pediatric intensive care unit, the PICU. Often parents
become emotional when we start to introduce ourselves as pediatric neurosurgeons, and it can be hard to stay on point when you
know that most everything coming out of your mouth is extremely
difficult for them to hear. Not hard in a "your most recent work peer
evaluations are not ideal" kind of way, but hard in a "please someone wake me up from this terrible dream" kind of way.

I remember meeting two-year-old Allie in the PICU several years
ago. She was lying flat and immobile in the ICU bed, the ventilator
hissing its regulated, even breaths for her. Apparently, she had been
completely healthy until her mom had noticed that she was weak in
the left leg while playing in the backyard, just the slightest amount.
Soon, she was unable to move the leg at all. Quickly they were off
to the ER, then for emergency brain imaging and the unstoppable
descent into their family's new nightmare.

Now nurses moved around her bed quickly, adjusting drips and silencing the occasional alarming monitor. Allie was comatose, unresponsive to all but the deepest stimulation. Her parents stood stunned just off to the side at the head of the bed, holding her hand and staring at their daughter, who was as close to death as they had ever seen anyone. Moments before meeting them, I had looked at her brain MRI with my resident and Haley Vance, my phenomenal nurse practitioner partner. She and I have worked together for fifteen years now, and she really is one of the main reasons our team is so successful. I remember telling them both before we walked in the room that it was not the image of a child who would do well, perhaps a 5 percent chance of survival at best. I could not help but begin to think of the difficult conversation to come.

Her brain MRI showed a large bleed in her brainstem, the pons specifically. The normal brain was compressed from the inside out, the pontine brain tissue now only a thin rim displaced by the blood clot, most likely from a hemorrhagic cavernous malformation. It was gigantic considering the small space. At that point in my career, I had never seen a hemorrhage quite that large in that part of the brain with the patient still alive. The brainstem, as detailed earlier, is a small space with a great deal going on. Not ideal to have a large blood clot in the center of it all.

The parents were called directly by their pediatrician while Allie was still in the scanner to relay to them what the radiologist was seeing on the initial images. When the MRI was finally completed, she was taken directly back up to the PICU, and our team met them there, learned her recent history, examined her, and called me.

"Hello, I'm Dr. Wellons, one of the pediatric neurosurgeons," I said as I walked up to the bedside to examine her. "I'm so sorry to be telling you this. Your daughter is very sick. I know that you know that. She's had some bleeding inside her brain, a stroke of sorts, and it's in a very important place."

"Can you take it out?" the dad said. He looked exhausted. They both did. I could imagine how little sleep they must have been going on. "It's a stroke? She's only two. Are you sure?" His questions were starting to come rapid-fire.

There's a pause that comes when I have to confirm to parents what they know, or suspect: that their child is close to death. In the seconds before the words come, I am acutely aware that their lives will be forever changed. There is no effective way to mitigate the pain and deliver what must be said. I remind myself that they are this child's parents. They have loved her and cared for her, and they need to know what is happening. It does not matter that I don't want to tell them. It does not matter that I know deeply in my own chest that I could not bear the news if someone was telling it to me. They need to understand. It is my job.

"Well," I replied. "Some strokes are from not enough blood flow, and some are from too much."

"Is she going to live?" her mom asked.

"She's very sick, and I am concerned that she may not make it through this," I said and then paused again.

"But she may," the mother said, looking up at me, "make it through this . . ." Her last words trailed off.

"She could," I said. "There is always a chance."

And I left it at that.

"So it's a stroke now? I thought it was a brain tumor," the father said, rubbing his temples with his fingers. "Somebody else said it was a brain tumor."

"Well, I don't think it's that," I said softly. "It looks to me like a blood vessel malformation." It's so hard to know how to describe this to people. The word "malformation" sounds so clinical and distant, like the "abnormality on the X-ray" or "your family member just expired."

"What do you mean, 'malformation'?"

"It's a collection of little abnormal"—*damn that word*—"blood pockets, like veins, but they can bleed and cause major problems in the brain," I said. "Problems like what your daughter's going through."

"So it's not cancer?"

"No, I don't think it's cancer." As I said this, they pulled each other closer, side by side.

"Thank you, Doctor," they said.

"But I've not done anything. In fact, I really can't do anything now because she's too sick to take to the operating room in her current state and it's deep in the brain and we have to see if she will survive in order to . . ." It was my turn to be rapid-fire. I was rambling the news out, as if it didn't take the first time I said it to them and I needed to make it very clear.

The mom cut in: "Our Allie's a fighter, Doctor. She's going to get better." Then she turned back toward her daughter, her discussion with me clearly done. Her husband nodded. It was time for me to go.

Indeed, over the next few months and against all odds, Allie did stabilize. Gradually, she began to improve. Weeks of inpatient rehab followed by outpatient rehab. All the while, the blood around the malformation resorbed. It shrank slightly. At that point, perhaps she would never need surgery. Even I began to believe it.

Then, suddenly, another bleed. This time not as severe as the last, but the lesion had expanded again. She wasn't as neurologically affected as the last time, but this was likely a sign of things to come. Another bleed like the initial one would be tough for her to survive. Neither radiation nor chemotherapy would be effective. Radiation has not shown to be effective in treating these types of vascular lesions, and chemotherapy is reserved for brain tumors. It was to be surgery or to let the natural history play out, meaning she lives as she is and her parents know at any time the bottom could drop out.

It became time for a go/no-go decision regarding the operating room. Cavernous malformations that are down deep in the brainstem like this are challenging to remove. Particularly those in the middle of the pons. To get to the lesion, we would have to enter from the back of the brain. The only way to do that is to traverse the floor of the fourth ventricle, the equivalent of the neurosurgical no-man's-land, a minefield of important brainstem nuclei and tracts. Some of these cavernous malformations grow closer to the sides or the front of the brainstem, and approaches from those directions involve drilling away part of the base of the skull in order to get there. I've done them before; often the drilling takes longer than the resection, but that would be of no help here. The lesion came up just underneath the floor; it was where the rim was thinnest. The question came to me again: Should we let her bleed a third time? Or move forward with resection, knowing that there would be a cost to getting it out. I did not think she could survive another bleed. I believed it was time to take it out. The parents were in agreement. Plans were made to move ahead.

The floor of the fourth ventricle looks, oddly enough, like a kite, a standard diamond-shaped kid's kite. The upper reaches are smaller, hidden up under the superior cerebellar peduncles, structures that look like the angled walls in the top floor of a house but that carry information running to and from the cerebellum and are responsible for coordination. Above all of that is the cerebellum itself, responsible for all coordination in the body. The lower portion of the floor is divided from the top by a series of long neurons running along the short axis; from east to west, called the stria medullaris. The midline spar of the kite is the median sulcus and divides one side from the other. But the lower portion holds several key nuclei that are responsible for swallowing, breathing, nausea, tongue movement, and alertness level. Right above the stria is a small bump called the facial colliculus. This is where the facial nerve coming from deeper in the pons runs up and around the sixth nerve nucleus, responsible for lateral eye movement. It's a key landmark in surgery, and damage directly to that area takes out facial movement on that side of the face as well as lateral eye movement. In addition, this particular minefield in Allie is squashed out to the sides from the internal hemorrhage. The approach to lesions in this area is in a small zone one centimeter above the facial colliculus and five millimeters over toward the peduncle wall. Taking out something like this is like taking a large walnut out through a small keyhole. Except the walnut is full of blood and everything around it is important for Allie to be able to interact with the world around her.

In the OR, she lay prone on the operating table, her head clamped in a vise of sorts that keeps the head still. (It's put on after the patient is fully anesthetized.) The back of her head was prepped and draped and the skin opened straight down the midline. We divide the upper neck muscles and temporarily remove a sizable piece of skull to give us the angle that we need to get the cavernous malformation out through the planned opening. Once the dura is open and the cerebellar hemispheres are gently retracted out to either side, we bring the operating microscope in. The kite is in full view as the "real part" of the operation begins despite it being ninety minutes since we cut skin. In order for us to tell where to enter the brainstem—meaning, cut into it with a microscopic sharp knife—we stimulate the floor of the fourth ventricle with a slight electrical current until the tiny needles we have in the facial muscles detect a twitch, telling us where the facial colliculus and tract are as they move through the pons to exit laterally into the temporal bone.

Then, using the tiny knife, we are through the floor, and immediately dark blue blood begins to pour out, the liquefied blood clot extruding through the hole. Our monitoring holds steady. Then we begin the dissection within the venous pockets, carefully removing them one by one. As we do this, the heart rate begins to swing wildly. We stop to let things settle, then start again. Over and over. Stopping. Starting again. We keep an important engorged internal vein intact that would cause her to stroke even worse if we damaged it. Before we know it, five hours have passed under the microscope and we are done.

I look down to see a cleft in the floor of the fourth ventricle that is clearly larger than a keyhole, unavoidable based on the lesion size. *Is it possible to have done this without further cost?* I hope to myself. Doubt creeps in. *Was this the right decision?* I veer off into that place we are supposed to avoid as pediatric neurosurgeons. Not introspection, that place is critical. But the place of self-doubt that can paralyze you in the middle of a challenging operation. An operation that needs to be done to stop the bleeding, to take out the tumor, or to bring that child back from over the edge. I pull it back together and work a bit longer under the microscope. Then we are done and we start to close up and Allie begins the long road of recovery.

After more than seven years from the events that have forever changed her life, Allie continues to recover. She's back in school with her friends but debilitated. Her words are stilted and slow to come at times. Her movement is choppy and she uses an upright walker to get herself around. But she has come a long way from being comatose and on a ventilator. In the time between then and now, she navigated another, similar surgery for a small recurrence of the cavernous malformation. This time behind that normal vein we worked so hard to keep intact. It again took her months to recover, but she did, once again walking into my clinic and sitting herself down in the examination chair. After that, a small plate used to secure the bone flap back to her skull wore through her skin. We removed that in a thirty-minute procedure, and she went home the same day. Allie was *amazed* that could happen, even asking me at the follow-up clinic visit why I didn't let her go home the same day after the other operations. Several months later, she began to slowly decline, her walking a little less vigorous, conversations less spontaneous. A follow-up MRI showed that she had developed hydrocephalus. We performed a procedure called an endoscopic third ventriculostomy, which bypasses the CSF blockage internally in lieu of a shunt. Then she was back on track to recovery again. Recently, she slowed down again, and her hydrocephalus had returned. We repeated the procedure, and again she's right back to it.

I mentioned to her mother, Carolyn, at a recent clinic visit how phenomenally resilient I thought their daughter was. How each time she bounced back from surgery, I was amazed at her strength. During the time in which I was facing and recovering from the muscle tumor in my upper leg and pelvis, I found *myself* drawing from memories of *her* and *her resilience,* as well as others I had taken care of along the way. I was floored by my own existential threat of a tumor, and this little girl faced a similar fate head-on. Allie had lived through challenges that many of us would never have to navigate our entire lives. Each time, she was back to the stand-up walker, back to speech therapy, back to school.

"What is it about her that enables her to do this?" I asked Carolyn. What is it like to see your nine-year-old daughter go through so much yet somehow push through it?

"This is all she's ever known," Carolyn answered. "We knew her before all of this and she was early to walk, early to babble, frustrated to not be understood clearly even at that age. She was always pushing. But her bleed happened when she was two. Now this is her normal. It's all she's really ever known. Her entire life has been one recovery after another."

I watched as Allie stood herself up, wobbling just a little. Her mom put her hand out to steady her, but Allie pushed it away.

"M-o-m," she said slowly in a way that clearly meant *do not help me.*

"Dr. Wellons," Carolyn continued, nonplussed. "Do you remember at the very beginning, that very first time we met you when you explained to us what had happened and we said that Allie was a fighter?"

"I do," I replied. "She was comatose and hadn't started to recover at all. In fact, some of the hardest days were yet to come for all of you. I hadn't the foggiest idea how much of that to really convey. So, I kind of didn't."

"No, no you didn't. That was obvious," she said, laughing.

I laughed with her. Although I was only around at the most intense times, I felt as if I had walked a journey with their family. We watched as Allie was making her way to the clinic room door, then into the hall to go get a cartoon sticker from the nurses. She pushed her walker through the door frame, banging the door as she went, clearly with an intention of being somewhere else. Carolyn and I laughed together again. Then she looked up at me, her face immediately serious. All of a sudden I saw her at Allie's bedside years ago, holding her daughter's hand, her world having crashed down around her.

"That day you did something that I don't think you really realize. We've never told you."

She paused as she watched her once near-death daughter clatter down the hall to collect her sticker. I turned to face Carolyn. I had come to admire her and her family a great deal over the years. I braced myself slightly, not knowing what her next words would be.

"You may have thought that you were giving us the worst news of our lives. But we were living that when you walked in that night. What you did was give us hope. Hope that we've never, ever let go."

12

November-5411-Yankee

OVER THE END-OF-THE-YEAR holiday break in my second year of medical school, my family decided to eschew the comfort, familiarity, and tradition of the southern Mississippi family home to take up a friend's generous offer and relax for a week on Little Cayman Island over Christmas vacation. My own nuclear family at the time consisted of my parents and two older sisters. As time went by, husbands, boyfriends, and my own soon-to-be fiancée, Melissa, were added to our lives and the holiday trip. Sun, we were promised, surf, wind, and all that a wintered-out, sun-starved group could imagine, and it sounded like paradise. The week actually on Little Cayman was all that was promised and more. What was not promised, what none of us could have known or even imagined, were the events of the journey that got us there.

My father had been a pilot for twenty-five years before I was born, getting not only his driver's license in Mississippi at the age of fifteen but his pilot's license as well. In a story that had been repeated to me ad nauseam over the course of my life up to then, he had saved up enough money working in his father's dry cleaners as a child that he bought a small used Piper Cub soon after getting his license. That solidified a lifelong love affair with the sky, one that sustained him in ways none of us would ever truly understand beyond how fulfilled we saw it make him when we were with him.

In college, he entered flight school and ultimately the Air National Guard, rising over the course of a more than forty-year career to the retirement rank of major general. In between those bookends was a life of pushing high-performance fighters to their edge or leading transport crews on long-haul missions on the traditional National Guard weekends and two-week trips, some resulting in outlandish gifts from faraway places—that fishing buoy from Japan, an intricate folding screen from India, and several beautiful kites from Ecuador, among others.

Outside the military flying, a significant proportion of every waking weekend hour not in his work or home office was focused on flight in some way. He would on occasion fly a shared Cessna 172 to see his own mother near Pensacola with one of us—usually me—flying in the right-hand seat. I can remember him telling me in grade school to have my multiplication tables memorized by the wheels-up time or I couldn't go with him. When I did not quite have the higher 11s and 12s, he sat with me and quizzed me on the tarmac with the propeller spinning until I could repeat the entire table from memory. He would walk around the hangar at the local unmanned airstrip in our tiny hometown to look over the local planes, or head to the nearby town's municipal airport to check the company twin-engine plane that he still loved to fly. He refused to hire a pilot for his own trips, figuring he could get two things done at once: his work as president of the company and logging pilot hours.

At the time of the Little Cayman trip, I had 4.3 hours of official piloting (that is, with an instructor who was not my father) in a Cessna 152. In taking lessons earlier that summer, mostly due to the time spent in the air with him over the course of my life, I had pretty quickly worked my way through taking off, communicating on the radio, and setting the navigation (in the days before GPS) and had just started on the more formal aspects of landing on runways with traffic instead of grass strips. At any rate, my father decided he would fly four of us down to Little Cayman, including Melissa and me. We flew in a Piper Aztec, a twin-engine plane nicknamed the Aztruck due to its notoriety in the hauling of immense loads and bare-bones instrumentation. (Truly notorious, my father would tell me later, for smuggling marijuana into the States.) I would fly in the co-pilot seat, pulling my usual grueling duty of saying "Check."

"Flaps" . . . "Check."
"Control yoke free" . . . "Check."
"Fuel mixture rich" . . . "Check."

I counted around seventy-five "checks" of some type during one preflight. I was convinced as a child that he added more of them to see if I was paying attention or teach me some sort of lesson (which I couldn't figure out at the time but as a surgeon makes perfect sense now).

Once out of Miami, the highlight of the three-hour trip nearly due south would be a climb to eight thousand feet in order to pass safely over Cuba. Interestingly enough, routing your flight path over Cuba must follow certain predetermined, for the lack of a better word, "highways" in the sky. Different planes fly at multitudes of different altitudes separated by five hundred or a thousand feet. To fly over Cuba in the 1990s, all of these "highways" in the sky converged at one spot on the map, the north side of the island across from Cayo Largo. At this point, all non-Cuban flights must assume at least eight thousand feet to be free from Cuban air, fly straight south all the while listening to a furious chatter of Cuban transmissions on the radio, and upon reaching the far point at the southern coast, over Cayo Largo itself, divert back to the predetermined route. Safely traversing the island nation, we pointed the Aztec toward Grand Cayman (the next point on our flight route) and activated the autopilot.

Nearly at the exact halfway point between the last Cuban marker and Grand Cayman, my father began to tap on the battery charge

gauge, not unlike the way in which we all tap our car's gas tank display when we know what we are reading couldn't possibly be correct. This gauge details if your battery is charging or if it is draining.
If the engine is off and you are on the ground warming the plane up
or if you are at low speeds at low altitudes, it is draining. If the airplane is in any other situation, it should be charging, or at least not
draining. The point at which I realized that the battery was indeed
draining was when the autopilot went out. At the moment in which
my father spoke into the radio to inform Havana of our problem,
our navigation went out, our radio died, and we experienced total
electrical failure.

This, needless to say, was not the most ideal of circumstances
to be in at this point. The three other passengers—Melissa; my oldest sister, Eve; and her boyfriend at the time, Steve—clearly notic-
ing the absence of digits in cockpit instruments and the significant
increase in discussion between my father and me, all began to look
around for life jackets not typically present on a twin-engine plane.
Instructing me to neither circumvent clouds nor deviate one-tenth
of a degree from our current compass heading, my father told me
to fly the plane as he dug around in his bags for something. I would
suppose over the years I could occasionally be a bit of an unruly
son, giving my father fits once in a while and countering his opin-
ions on more than one occasion. I had felt little option in going into
medicine, somehow purposefully positioned into it over time as if
he had whispered it into my ear as I slept as a young boy. I was still
coming to terms with postcollege adulthood and this new life as a
medical student.

It was then, however, that I briefly transformed into the ideal son.
More "Yes, sirs" came from my mouth than during all the speeding
tickets and work ethic speeches I had received from him combined.
After a minor eternity of digging, he produced a handheld, battery-
operated, two-way radio that he had acquired only three weeks
prior to our flight. Its sales tag still hung from its imitation leather

case. Using an antenna cord found in the aeronautical equivalent of the Aztec's glove compartment, he then spliced the cord to the airplane's antenna via an input terminal normally used for our headsets and microphones. With this setup he then attempted to contact Havana to no avail. Either the battery's power was insufficient, or they simply chose not to respond.

By now I had reviewed my 4.3 hours of formal instruction nearly four hundred times in my head and was applying it wholeheartedly to my task at hand. The clouds were beneath us—at around three thousand feet—so we were relatively free from significant turbulence. We had really no exact idea of our present position, other than an extrapolation from our last known instrument heading. Two degrees off proper course would take us out of visual and rapidly dying radio range of our target. If we were to pass it even farther to the east or west, we could possibly be out of the Grand Cayman airport's radar range if our change was drastic enough. Our fuel supply could ill-afford any situation keeping us in the air much longer if we had indeed strayed. The low clouds formed another barrier to visual contact, but a drop too far down could limit our glide distance in the case of further malfunction.

Finally, an American Airlines DC-10 flying toward Miami at thirty-five thousand feet above us responded. Upon hearing my father, the captain identified himself.

"November-5411-Yankee"—our airplane's identification number—"seems you're in a bit of a bind," he stated.

They radioed our status to Havana, who did absolutely nothing but steer us to the frequency for Grand Cayman.

"Desperate situation," we heard the captain tell the Cuban air controllers.

"Contact radio frequency 120.2."

"Need radar location."

"Contact 120.2."

The captain reassured us that he had radioed our general position and situation back to Grand Cayman (in case we had to ditch *in the ocean*, I realized without his saying it).

As the captain's voice crackled into static, Dad started the automatic familiar rhythm of SOS on the radio. The dots and dashes pervaded the cabin. I looked back at Melissa, who was wide-eyed and mouthed to me, "Is it always like this with your family?" Then Dad informed me that if we did not locate the island in four minutes, we would have to turn around and land in Cuba. The idea of spending part of my well-deserved medical school vacation detained in Cuba did not appeal to me. At this point, HBO-instilled visions of gun beatings and American taunting welled up within me.

Two weeks before, there had been a newsworthy event where one recently defected father (who just happened to take a MiG with him when he left Cuba) landed on a crowded highway in a borrowed Cessna 150, loaded his family, and made a getaway while the Cuban Air Force was scrambling. Needless to say, this was not a time of great communication between the two countries. Equally unpalatable was the concept of dashing under the radar to the American-owned naval base, Guantánamo Bay, where Dad assured me he could talk us down before they started shooting. (*Sure*, I thought, *if we still have a working radio.*) I shook my head to focus and rededicated myself to the dual task of flying and scanning the water for any sign of land whatsoever.

Ironic, I thought, to find myself somewhere over the Caribbean Sea south of Cuba looking for a place to land with a rapidly depleting amount of fuel and piloting something nicknamed an Aztruck used most famously for hauling pot.

The onboard clock had died with the electricity, but my watch indicated nearly an hour had passed since total outage occurred. Time was running out. We peered down through the clouds and waited for any opening.

"Dad, I think I see something," I said.

"Well, son," he said matter-of-factly, "if it's land, then by all means fly toward it."

"Never mind, it's just a sailboat . . ."

I started to look away but stopped. *A sailboat,* I thought. *Where there are sailboats, there is usually . . .*

"LAND," I ecstatically yelled out as right then a hole had opened up in the clouds just big enough to make out lush solid-green land. Without hesitation I dove for it.

Recounting the story to friends later, I would barrel roll my hand like Pappy Boyington in his World War II Corsair rolling out of the sun to wreak havoc on an unsuspecting squadron of Japanese Zeros. The rapid decrease in altitude brought us into radio contact with the already frantic Grand Cayman air traffic controllers.

"Come in, November-5411-Yankee . . . come in, November-5411-Yankee . . ."

"This is November-5411-Yankee," we responded. "Go ahead."

"Oh, mon, we got da whole island hearing bout dis one. What is your status, mon? Are you still without power?" The faint sounds of reggae played in the background. I honestly imagined them waving marijuana smoke away and sitting up when they heard us respond.

"Roger, tower. No power," my father replied, face set. "But we have two engines working. Request flyby to verify landing gear deployment."

"Sure, sure, mon. Tank God! How many souls on board?"

I chuckled as a smile finally crept across my father's face.

"Five souls . . . repeat five souls on board," he spoke back into the belly of the now nearly drained radio.

I gladly relinquished my duties to him, although it was quite difficult to remove my hands from the control yoke where the tightness of my grip had formed a near vacuum. He performed the flyby with the belly of the plane rolled up slightly so the tower could tell us the status of our landing gear. It had not come down. So, he instructed me on how to pump it down using a lever just next to my feet, which I did for the very first and last time of my life to date. Soon afterward, he had performed a perfect landing, during which, to our relief, the landing gear held. We taxied over to the terminal and pulled up to a ground crewman, who chucked our wheels as if nothing had happened, as if moments before we weren't considering ditching in the Caribbean Sea.

The remainder of the afternoon was spent explaining our story to the curious officials of the Grand Cayman airport and fixing the plane. The problem had been a malfunction of the alternator and was rectified with a new wire and smiling mechanic by the morning. We spent a night of eating, drinking, and laughing as we came to terms with what had happened. I remember sitting at the table that night drinking a beer with my father. Something we had done before but in not quite the same way. On this night, we clinked the bottles together in a toast and drank deeply. He laughed loudly, telling stories of other adventures in the air. I didn't know it at the time, but it was then I learned about grace under pressure. I knew that I would never see him in the same way after that day, and I didn't. He had been a man larger than life with experiences I could only make up in my head. This time I had sat beside him in a crisis, flown alongside him, and calmly worked up a solution with him. He had needed me that day, perhaps truly for the first time, I thought, and I realized how desperately I had needed for him to.

The next day, we made the thirty-minute jump flight to Little Cayman, bringing groceries for the week and a grateful family finally to our intended destination. That quick flight was joyous, our hands smoothly moving together over the controls, the familiar sight of functioning instrumentation now back. I knew even then that I was forever changed by the events of the prior twenty-four hours. Gone would be the days of quietly pushing against my father in order to better define myself, who I felt I was, how I wanted to move through this life on my own, as I had for many of the years before. I relinquished the pushback that I carried with me into medical school. All of that just dropped away. Those months to follow would become my favorite time with him, by far the most meaningful.

Right then, side by side in that cockpit laughing as we did a flyby to scout the unmarked grass-and-dirt landing strip unfolding beneath us, I was equally certain that we had all our lives ahead of us, an endless reservoir of time. The bright sun rose behind us to the east as we came around and lined up for the final approach. There was no tower to talk to, so once we looked around to establish visual confirmation of clear skies, we just simply talked to ourselves. As we throttled back the engines, our airspeed dropped. The nose gently tipped down in response. Beneath us the trees moving past rapidly turned to scrub and the scrub turned to grass; then it was only the worn strip below. We were gliding our way in, nearly silent at this point. One of us, I no longer can remember who, brought the nose back up just enough as we leveled out with the field on both sides of us, and before I even realized it, we had touched down, safely back to earth once again.

—•—

13

Anger

T HREE HUNDRED AGAIN! Clear!"

The patient, now only partially draped for surgery, convulsed as the electricity from the cardioversion paddles surged through her body. The towel loosely covering her neck wound somehow remained in place.

No change. Still in V-fib. Not a heart rhythm compatible with life. The monitor alarm came back on.

"Turn it up to 360 joules now!" I said, much louder than was necessary. "Clear!"

Again, she convulsed.

Nothing.

"Again! Clear!"

This time, however, after the shock passed through her, the monitor began to trace and sound out a pulse. Her heart rhythm returned.

"Sinus rhythm!" said a voice standing at the head of the OR bed.

"Oh, *hell* yes," said the male scrub tech standing across from me. Both of us were still fully gowned and gloved. His instrument set was slung back toward the wall, a portion of it on the floor having fallen there in a loud clatter in the first few movements after everyone realized our patient's heart had stopped.

I looked down and saw slight red burns outlined on my patient's chest where the paddles had initially made contact during the first shock. In my initial excitement of tearing down the surgical drapes, I had forgotten to put conducting gel on the cardioversion paddles. A rookie move for a *relatively* experienced senior resident until the on-the-ball circulating nurse quickly found some conducting gel for us to use.

This is nothing like TV, I thought to myself, thinking of the confident way people on medical TV shows slam those paddles together with gel and make the circular motion with them before inevitably shocking someone back into the conversation they were just having.

I looked up at the now steady rhythm on the OR monitor. Her blood pressure was coming up in a good way. I realized that each and every face in that OR was staring at me, awaiting my next word.

"Um, nice work, everyone," I stumbled out. "MJ, thanks for the gel."

Lying on the OR table just below me was the fiftyish-year-old woman we had just shocked back to life. The towel over the hastily clamped-shut wound on her neck was starting to stain with blood. Now that her circulation was restored, everything we didn't close in the midst of the emergency had started to bleed. Minutes before I had been dissecting past the strap-like sternocleidomastoid muscle of the lateral neck and was well on my way through the carotid sheath in order to isolate her carotid artery. Once that was exposed and ready, my attending was to come back in, and he and I were to perform a carotid endarterectomy, just as we had done twenty times before that one. I had come to enjoy the procedure. I found that it was quick and neat and seemed to have a huge positive impact on patients in the long run.

The procedure, done for more than thirty years, restores adequate blood flow to the brain and, along with blood thinners, helps to prevent stroke, especially a first stroke. The carotid endarterectomy itself has been studied more than almost any other surgical procedure over the years. Data exists that dictates when to perform it, who should perform it, and now when to use newer technology to stent it open from the inside. There are variations of the procedure, depending on the specialty performing the surgery. Studies exist indicating whether to sew in a patch to expand the artery or not after carefully removing the cholesterol and calcified plaque from inside the carotid wall, or to use a shunt during the procedure to bypass the clamped vessel during the repair and keep blood flowing to the brain. Even whether or not using an operating microscope reduces the likelihood of postoperative stroke. All battled out in academic societies and journals over the years by vascular surgeons, neurosurgeons, cardiovascular surgeons, and cardiologists. That war, among others, rages on.

But here, away from all of that, we had this one woman with clamps holding her wound together, a thousand tiny places bleeding, and no endarterectomy done. What to do? I held pressure and stalled until my attending made it back to the room.

"What the flying hell is going on?" he said as he came in near breathless.

We explained the whole story, at least what we could piece together. As I moved through prepping, draping, and opening the neck, all was going well. Her heart tracing was normal. Then, suddenly, her T wave widened until it fully flipped (which signifies lack of adequate blood flow to the heart) and then ventricular tachycardia—V-tach—and then full-on fibrillation. After a few seconds of his looking up at the monitor to see that her rhythm had normalized, his answer was for me to close the woman up and get her to the cardiologists as soon as possible.

"What about the caro—" I began to ask.

"Never mind that," he said. "You just had to shock her four times to get a rhythm back. Just get cardiology to see what is going on with her heart."

Once I had her closed up appropriately, she was taken to the cardiology "cath lab," where heart angiograms are done. An angiogram can be done for nearly any organ, most commonly the heart and nowadays a not-as-distant-as-it-used-to-be second, the brain. In the cardiac cath lab, she underwent stent placement in several constricted areas in her coronary vessels, previously unknown because she had been symptom free when asked prior to the operation. After a long and eventful day, she made it to the ICU, where she would need to recover in preparation for another attempt at surgery down the line. Her cardiologist sat at the nurses' station, his cowboy boots propped up on the chair next to him as he wrote his post-procedure note. He filled me in on the events in the cath lab and told me that he had spoken with the family.

Her family, a husband around a decade her senior and two sons, who looked to be in their early twenties, took none of this news well. They were angry. Angry at us surgeons. Angry at the anesthesiologists. Angry at the cardiologists. Angry at the whole system. It took some time talking them down that night, but finally we were able to persuade them to head to a nearby hotel for sleep. The hospital would cover the costs. Over the next several days, they remained distant, as if they were plotting their next move. I had heard they took photographs of her chest where the singe from the initial shock in the OR was fading. All of it unfortunate and particularly astonishing to me since we had been able to bring their wife and mother back from the brink.

"Why aren't they more grateful?" I asked my attending. This was the first time I had seen this type of raw emotion in a patient's family so up close.

"Well, she's not through it yet. There's a great deal of stress added when you think you or your family is going to be through something but then they are not. People handle uncertainty in different ways. Some come to the table with little trust for the medical system, just like this family when I met them in clinic the first time," he continued. "Don't take it personally. You really need to cut them some slack."

With that insight and advice, I began to actively seek them out to explain things after rounds. This seemed to ease their minds a bit, even taking the time to learn my name and role in her care. After a few days of amiable communication, I sat down and explained again all that had happened since the aborted surgery and why we needed to proceed. The plan was to move forward in two days. All the teams agreed that she needed to get that carotid stenosis taken care of. The patient herself was quiet and trusting. She asked few questions.

"I trust you all," she said, smiling. "You brought me back once already."

My attending and I were in the operating room with another patient for a good bit of the next day. That particular case—a craniotomy for a deep-seated brain tumor—had started around noon. It was evening when we realized that we were done. Time moves differently when the mind is focused. We were, frankly, quite pleased with ourselves, just starting to close up. Music played in the background when the urgent call came.

Our carotid patient was coding again.

I scrubbed out and ran to the unit. The ICU team there was actively coding her. She had been intubated and was lying unresponsive on her back in the bed. Someone was intermittently performing chest compressions. This time there was no bringing her back. The monitor never started back up any type of rhythm the entire time, regardless of shock or medicine administered. One moment she was fine eating her dinner. The next she was unresponsive in V-fib and finally terminal asystole.

I knew immediately that I had to find her family. I looked around the ICU waiting room and then tried to call them. No answer at the room in the hotel. I headed back to the OR to help finish up the craniotomy.

Just over an hour later we were done with the closure. (For the record, it takes some time to get the dura closed, the bone replaced, and the layers of the scalp put back together with multiple sutures.) I took the patient up to the ICU, spoke to that family, and again looked around for the other patient's family. Still nowhere to be found. Finally, after what I felt was an exhaustive search, I headed to the locker room to change and start the process of getting out of the hospital. I would need to check on the rest of our patients and make sure no more orders needed to be written. By 10:00 P.M., I was walking out.

That's when I saw the patient's family coming toward me from the other end of the long hall to the parking lot. It was late, so the hall was otherwise empty, *and isolated,* I realized. I could see the red exit sign at the end, the doors propped open, and the dark square leading out into the parking lot just past them. When they saw me, they started to run toward me.

I briefly remember thinking that I needed to make sure they knew what had happened.

"You son of a *bitch!*" one shouted at me as they approached.

Oh crap, I thought.

Quickly, they were in front of me.

"I'm so very sorry," I said. "I'm afraid she died a little while . . ."

"We know she's dead, you son of a bitch." The husband and his sons surrounded me.

I remember talking quickly. I remember apologizing profusely. Then I remember running away as fast as I could down the hall into the darkness.

At some point later I sat in my car two blocks away from the hospital. I thought about how we had saved her the first time; then, despite all that was done afterward, she still died. I was angry. Angry that she died. Angry at that family for blaming me. For circling around me. *What was their plan?*

I slammed my fists onto the steering wheel. *To hell with them.*

I drove home, where my wife was already in bed, like a thousand other nights of my residency. Even rotating at the nearby private hospital, I still rarely made it home before 9:00 P.M. I rolled into bed and slept, fitfully. At one point I heard a car door slam and welcomed whatever they planned to do to me.

The next morning at 6:00, I arrived at work, the events of the previous night fresh on my mind, this day blurring into the last. The very first person I met on the way in was the boot-wearing cardiologist who had tried to save our patient with the multiple stents.

"Did you hear what happened last night?" he asked me.

I started to tell him how that family had surrounded me. How I had felt in danger and had run away.

How I had never felt that from a patient's family before, but he interrupted me.

"No, no, not that," he said.

He waved me off. "They walked into an active OR."

"Wait, what?" I said, dumbfounded. "They walked, fully clothed and unmasked, into an ongoing orthopedic operation. A freakin' femur for God's sake. And you know what they were yelling right before the security guard pulled them out?"

I was speechless. This would have been just after they confronted me.

"'Is this the place where they kill people?' That's what they were yelling as they pulled them out."

Death is unfathomable, whether you understand the physical processes that cause it or not. As our deepest mystery, it is not surprising that acceptance is impossible for some people. It is difficult for me to accept. But until that night, I had never experienced rage before. And from that point on, I have never underestimated the sometimes violent storm of emotions that can be displayed by family members in a time of stress. It is not always grief. Sometimes, it is anger and hate. Later in my career, I would come to be cyberbullied, and have my medical license investigated by an upset parent (and ultimately cleared). I even received a threat that something destructive would happen to my clinic. But none of it was like that very first night when I was alone and surrounded by that angry family in that long dark hall who wanted revenge for the death of their wife and mother, and my realization that my white coat, my "status," and my mistaken sense of untouchability were as weak as words, bestowing absolutely zero protection from the passions of man.

—————

14

Bucket Lines

A
LL SURGEONS HAVE mentors. And sometimes, when you find yourself in a tight spot, it is the wise words of your mentor that come to mind most clearly and save you.

One of my most notable mentors during residency training at Duke was a freshly minted pediatric neurosurgeon named Tim George. At the time, Tim had recently completed his own training, and Duke was his first faculty position. It was quickly clear to all of the residents that he was a talented surgeon and excellent communicator. He elevated everyone around him. His patients certainly loved him, as did his OR staff. In particular, the healthcare workers who transported patients, sterilized the equipment, and entered in the medical orders on the wards felt a great sense of commonality with him. Tim was a proud Black man who had grown up in Brooklyn (as he was quick to remind folks), and he loved the stark contrasts between his hometown and his new town in North Carolina. He also loved to contrast his upbringing in New York and mine in Mississippi (often mimicking me with a Foghorn Leghorn accent spoken during lulls in cases that nearly paralyzed us with laughter. *I say, I say, a-hand me that there a-hemostat. I'm just a simple country neurosurgeon, tryin' to get the day's work done*).

Tim brought a sense of calm and ease into the OR with him every morning that suffused the room. Given the energy in his OR and the high-intensity-stress wavelengths in the other ORs for the day, it was an easy decision for me on which room I wanted to be in. Operating on children was and is challenging; not only is the anatomy smaller and changing as a child grows, but the stress of the parents and caregivers around each case is as palpable as it is completely understandable. Somehow the OR environment that Tim created mitigated that stress just enough. During those training years as a fledgling neurosurgeon, you end up spending more time with stress than you ever thought possible, so any way to manage it is welcome.

In a single hour of being on call as a neurosurgical resident, you can sit with an elderly woman in the emergency department to tell her that the brain hemorrhage her husband of fifty years just suffered while shaving is not survivable and no surgery will change that. Then, just afterward, you can be called to the pediatric ICU to place a lifesaving drain in the brain of a four-year-old girl dying from elevated intracranial pressure and watch as the child opens her eyes a few minutes later, squeezing her parents' hands. One hour. In the span of one single hour, those things can happen. Over and over and over in the weeks, then months, then seven years of formal training. That job training, at least the part that deals in the intense and important human truths forged at the unspoken places we navigate, is never-ending.

Ultimately, one has no choice but to learn to live with stress. Taking every third day and night call rotation made it seem like you were always either on call, post-call, or getting ready to take call, which was indeed the case—for seven long years. Each beep of our pager would disrupt the flow of the operation, sometimes with a call back to the other party, be it trauma bay or ICU with a new emergency, or a nurse with a question, or a doctor with a consult. Regardless, one moment we were rapt in the intricate landscape of this new world we desperately wanted to learn to navigate, under the microscope or through the lens of an endoscope. The next, our attention was pulled away from the OR table to either relay an answer through the circulating nurse—leaning our heads awkwardly into the telephone receiver being held to the side of us while scrubbed, trying to get our ears on the receiver just so without contaminating ourselves—or, on occasion, to scrub out completely to manage a problem, taking us out of the OR indefinitely.

As a resident, managing the chaos of the world outside the OR taxed every part of my being. Rapid-fire crises will do that—six or seven things happening simultaneously, triaging them—ordering and managing by level of seriousness, thinking through each of them, quickly enough to avoid having more issues pile up. Over time, that processing became second nature, and certainly part of it was the clinical presentation of patients and the anxiety and sadness that it brought. It was always there. But we chose this field; we wanted to be neurosurgeons. The risk you take when you are often operating at the edge is that there are some patients you cannot pull back. The highs and lows of neurosurgery become near addictive over time. Mere sadness is not enough; it must be gut-wrenching grief. Frustration turns to disdain for anyone not trying as hard as you, and joy becomes heightened beyond what can be considered normal. Spending a few hours off with friends pales in comparison with getting to tell a wife that her husband will live and wake up and come home after all. *Thank you, Doctor. And thank you for all the sacrifices you have made along the way.*

These days the terms "burnout" and "moral injury" are used to describe the place that doctors and other healthcare workers with patient responsibility sometimes find themselves in. It's dangerous. Add a chronic lack of sleep and an environment of probing and second-guessing, and you can begin to lose trust in everyone around you. The constant beat of life-and-death decisions begins to change you in fundamental ways. Trust gives way to suspicion; care gives way to loathing. But back then we had no labels for this, just the anger. And the guilt.

As I think back to the 150-hour workweeks, the endless series of decisions asked of us, the confrontation and anger gradually replacing the compassion and care for our colleagues, it is clear to me that all of us as neurosurgery residents lived in that place back then.

Back then, amid all of it, I looked to Tim and saw someone who had made it out the other side with his humanity intact. He was a successful surgeon and had friends outside work, loved his family, and earnestly enjoyed being with his patients. As my residency years progressed, I had no idea if I could or would make it, but whatever the outcome I knew I wanted to have at least some of my humanity intact when I was done. Whatever Tim had, I wanted.

One particular morning on a day mid-residency, I had been assigned to Tim's OR by the chief resident, and I walked in for the first case of the day a few minutes late. I was distant, angry, and distracted. I had been ordered by the chief resident to "get myself together" after being on call the night before. But it didn't work. I slammed down my shoulder bag onto the floor next to the cabinet when there was no space left inside. Not an ideal state in which to do neurosurgery. There was a young OR tech who idealized Tim and liked working with the two of us and whom I liked a good bit, too. I somehow found myself almost at blows with him for something insignificant, the actual issue not memorable these many years later.

But the reason for my foul state has not left me. The night before, I had lost my first patient in the OR alone.

A twenty-five-year-old had been taken out by a stray falling bullet, fired into the sky by some excited reveler at an early-morning party. The bullet entered the top of his head and passed through the frontal lobe, slicing through the internal carotid artery as it passed through the cavernous sinus at the base of the skull, the former a major conduit for arterial blood under pressure directly from the heart, and the latter a confluence of vessels containing dark blue venous blood making its way back. During the emergency prepping of the head when I briefly stopped holding pressure in order to shave the hair, a geyser of blood shot up from the bullet hole. I would come to find out that the reason it was under such pressure was that it was jetting up from the severed artery at the base of the skull through the hole in his brain and out the top of his head.

Once the brain was exposed—a process that can take up to thirty minutes but in this case took three—I hastily placed two retractors normally reserved for the skin edges underneath the frontal lobe to expose the injury to the vessel. From such a small hole, the amount of blood was astounding. At times it sprayed up into my face and onto my surgical loupes. Holding pressure at the source didn't work. Stuffing it with balls of tight cotton didn't work. Blood kept pouring out, welling up and over the side of the craniotomy.

When I think of that night, the early lines from Tom Wolfe's *The Right Stuff* come to mind:

What do I do next? The mark of a good fighter pilot is that when all goes to shit, what is he yelling into his microphone? It isn't a prayer, it's: "I've tried A! I've tried B! I've tried C! I've tried D! Tell me what else I can try!"

After a futile final attempt to get just a single stitch into anything, blood pouring out all around my instruments up and over his frontal lobe, suddenly it was water in front of my eyes. One second red, then watery, then completely clear. He had bled out entirely while I tried in desperation to stop the bleeding. His circulating blood volume had been replaced by clear IV fluid. I became aware of the long uninterrupted sound of his flat line. I looked up to see that everyone else was still. I could not understand why they had stopped. At the end, the anesthesiologist had to pull me away, just like you see in the movies.

The attending neurosurgeon, on call as faculty for the night, never even had a chance to make it in, all of it had happened so fast. It was my very own first encounter with death without any extra layer protecting me from full responsibility. No attending surgeon. Just me, flailing away. *Tell me what else I can try!* It was a long way from glorious neurosurgery that I had idealized as a student glancing through that OR window. The nurses informed me that there was no family to talk to. No one had shown up with him. And no information about them. This was in the days before cell phones. No contacts to call. There was only this suddenly dead young man, killed by a stray bullet and my inability to stop the bleeding.

After he had been pronounced dead and his body transported out of the OR to the morgue, I walked into the empty locker room and peeled off my scrubs, sticky and wet where his blood had saturated through the protective surgical gown. I tossed my similarly soaked boxer shorts in the trash and showered there in the OR shower stall, watching as the thick blood coating my stomach, matting my pubic hair, and running down my thighs turned the shower floor red.

When I walked back into the OR later that morning, Tim could have easily dressed me down for being late or for having a terrible attitude. *Don't you know it's a privilege to operate!* Instead, while anesthesia placed the necessary IV lines for the operation, he took me out to the hall and asked what had happened. We sat down and he listened as I recounted the carnage from just a few hours before, and his head turned away as he remembered his own experiences and losses from his own training. We spoke for a few minutes, and when I was ready and with a hand on my shoulder, we started to walk back into the room to the next patient who needed our help.

"You gave that young man everything you had last night," he told me. "We cannot save every person in this OR. But we can try. And now there is an eight-year-old boy who needs your full attention."

Tim knew the way through this was to acknowledge the sadness and then to refocus on the next patient in front of you, on what we could do to help them. And we did that, together. It was the only way through. And I have repeated that over and over in the years since.

* * *

RECENTLY, WE BROUGHT a young girl up to the OR emergently. She had been shot, the circumstances unknown, and similar to years before, a jet of blood shot up from her head when the resident removed his hand. I recognized what it meant—a major blood vessel in the brain had been sheared off. She was close to death, her only chance was to get in quickly and stop the bleeding. It all happened first thing in the morning, 7:00. The very best team we had was prepping our main neurosurgery OR for an elective craniotomy, so the trays were open, the room ready, everyone was fully engaged. Other members of the neuro OR team came in to help open instruments. It was all hands on deck with a team that had been lauded over and over for their dedication.

But even all of this was not enough. We did our best to stop the bleeding, but her brain began to swell, massively, outside her opened skull. I was blindly placing aneurysm clips in an attempt to stop the bleeding jetting up from the depths. I knew then she would not survive, possibly not even making it off the table. Somehow, we were able to close up quickly and get her up to the PICU for the family to surround her bed and say goodbye. I left just as they began to file in. We had not saved her. There was no reason for me to inject myself even further into their grief.

When I returned to the OR, the entire team was silent, clearly affected by the loss they had just been a part of. Blood was being mopped from the floor, off the monitors around the room. Trays of used instruments were being removed. The room would soon be set up for the next operation, a teenager with severe life-limiting headaches and a Chiari I malformation; part of the brain was being compressed due to a malformation that was present at birth and had worsened. A successful surgery could bring his life back to normal.

I remembered that quiet time with Tim years before. I asked for everyone's attention in the room. Eight solemn sets of eyes looked up at me as they paused their work.

"She had the best team," I said.

The scrub nurse turned her head away as the tears began to fall.

I continued, "She had the best team, a team that could not have been more ready this morning. The circumstances could not have been better. But sometimes even that doesn't matter. Each and every one of you did your job to absolute perfection just now."

Tim's words came back to me: "We cannot save every person in this OR. But we can try."

I thought of that morning long ago when he looked past me to his own memories.

"So there is a child in holding right now who needs us," I continued. "We can make his life better once we are done. I can promise you that in the process of that, of helping to heal him, we ourselves will heal just enough to move on."

OVER THE YEARS, Tim and I would keep up from time to time; our families would mingle at various national meetings. We promised to get a beer one day, never quite getting it to work when we were rarely in the same city. Then a call came. Tim had suddenly and unexpectedly died. Way too early, in his late fifties. The news came to me from an old friend; he had been the one to volunteer to call me because everyone knew this would be a blow. Soon, phone calls and texts latticed out in our small pediatric neurosurgical community. Most of us knew that he had taken on endurance sports car racing as a hobby and had grown to be quite successful. While in the midst of a race, he radioed in that he was feeling unwell, then went radio silent. He was able to navigate off the track onto pit row, but was unresponsive as his car rolled to a stop, just past their designated spot. He was formally pronounced dead in a local emergency department. It was a tremendous blow to his family, his patients, the close-knit racing community in which he had existed, and our own field of pediatric neurosurgery.

Once I processed the tragic news, I quickly resolved to travel to his memorial service in Austin, Texas, where he had spent the last decade or so helping to build up the local medical school and children's hospital. As the time approached to leave, I found that the business of the intervening workdays distracted me enough that I had to stop and remind myself that I was not traveling to see him. I was traveling to say goodbye. Goodbye to a person who showed kindness and grace during that crucible of training, sometimes with a hand on the shoulder, a gentle redirection, or the hard answers when I would struggle, all so critically important early in a career.

On the flight to the service is when it occurred to me that there is a long list of people like Tim spanning back to my childhood who have handed me from one to the next, bucket line–like, to the present. I began to reflect on them a great deal, cultivating a sense of profound gratitude, from my parents to enthusiastic English litera-ture professors, skillful surgeons to influential department chairs. It is difficult to imagine life without these mentors along the way. Every step then self-actualized. The energy of activation vastly higher. The path less lit, more unsure.

But an unlit path is not my story, or the story of most of us in this field. All of those years of training to be a pediatric neurosurgeon gives us ample opportunities to find mentors, people we want to emulate . . . *Did you see him/her take out that tumor? Poetry!* . . . In our field, we spend so much time with our teachers, operating at their side, that it is nearly impossible to not tell their jokes, share their successes and failures, and live small parts of their lives. From all of that time together, you begin to know their kids and their spouses and, if you are lucky, catch a glimpse of the long bucket line span-ning back into their own past.

At the service, I learned that as a Black man in the 1960s and 1970s, Tim had had a bucket line that was much shorter than mine. I had never had any idea of this. Growing up in Brooklyn, he felt the rampant prejudice and near-immovable barriers inherent in our society for Black men and women, especially at that time. Yet, somehow, Tim willed himself into Columbia University, then NYU for medical school, Yale and Northwestern for his neurosurgery training, always persevering, pushing himself across the next gap in the line. His first job was at Duke as an assistant professor. Then, nearly a decade later, he left for Austin to help grow the children's hospital and the newly formed academic medical center there. Along the way, at every stop, he mentored countless students, residents, and junior faculty. Nothing was more meaningful to him than the work that he did for Black children interested in medicine. Over the years he would come to be honored time and time again for this.

I have been involved in resident education in one way or another for nearly twenty years as a faculty member across two institutions. Even after I stepped down as their program director, the residents still humor me on Saturday mornings after rounds as we drink coffee and I draw arrows and boxes on the whiteboard linking their pasts to their futures, each time returning to the topic of identifying mentors on their own career journey, to seek out those with admirable qualities or desirable skill sets to incorporate into a new self. The training hours may not be quite as long these days, but the moments to process are most certainly the same. Empathy from the teachers means the same now as it did then, and on occasion when I'm sitting with a resident helping her or him process a death, I cannot help but think of that morning when I would have unleashed whatever pent-up anger on anyone in my way.

Then someone sat with me and listened and focused me on what lay ahead. *Yes, this is hard, but we are needed. You must gather yourself.*

When I was a junior resident, that same man showed me how to pull the needle through the dura just so and re-clasp it for the next stitch. "Like this," he would say. Then he'd throw two of the most efficient and perfect suture passes, each time handing it back to me. Gradually, the teaching was in more advanced surgical skills, resecting an epileptic focus in the brain or closing a myelomeningocele or performing some other highly complex endeavor that over time becomes routine. The instructions matured as he matured me. "Keep that plane going between the tumor and white matter" or "Follow that feeding vessel farther out before you take it." If I didn't do it, then the teaching equivalent of two throws of the suture would occur. My surgical education advanced in these aliquots. Until one day, I was somewhere else, and it was only his voice I heard in my head as I operated.

I took out my first pediatric brain tumor with Tim, wrote my first academic paper with him, and followed him into pediatric neuro-surgery because I was drawn to who he was and how he did things. In the elective year in the middle of my residency, Tim would allow me to use his office at night and on the weekends to work on data-bases and write academic papers.

Those days in his office presaged the fact that clinical research would become a significant part of my career. A book about writing academic papers is profoundly less interesting than the stories of the children that we've been able to help, but it is important here to note: That first paper written with Tim years ago has turned into more than 250 academic papers. Some I'm proud of, some less so. Over time as I moved through this field, I realized there was a way to make an impact on a broader plane by learning more about neurosurgical problems on a population level. Thanks to patient and supportive partners, I was able to take one class at a time as an attending neurosurgeon and slowly obtain a master's degree in epidemiology. From that degree has come a whole aspect of my life focused on research based on race, socioeconomic status, and gender disparity in healthcare access for children with neurosurgical issues. I'm proud to help and promote work that narrows that gap, and I like to think that Tim would be pleased to know those early days of entrusting a mid-level resident with the keys to his office somehow continued his own mission to level the playing field and allow more and more bucket lines to form.

On one particular weekend, the top cabinet door above his desk was stuck partially open. There was an envelope caught in the door keeping it from closing. When I opened it, letter after letter and card after card poured out onto his desk—an avalanche of gratitude, grace delivered back to him. Each one, every single one, from a parent opening their heart in thanks. Or, in a child's handwriting: "To Dr. Tim George, my hero." And there would be the two of them as stick figures holding hands and smiling, the yellow sun in the upper corner and a bumpy rainbow arcing across the sky.

Just after my arrival in Nashville, before Tim's death, a young boy from an inner-city magnet school came with his mother to my academic office to interview me for his eighth-grade career day. As we were finishing up, he put down his pen, looked up from his notes, and, in as serious a tone as he could muster, asked me, "Dr. Jay, for real. Do you know any Black pediatric neurosurgeons?"

I pointed to a photo I have on my office wall behind him. It is of Tim and me operating together during my training, and it is still right in my line of sight when I sit at my desk.

"Yes, I do," I said. "His name is Tim George. He was my teacher and now he is my friend."

The boy's mouth dropped open in silence, and his mother began to cry. "You see, baby," she said, "you really can be anything you want to be."

15

---·•·---

Rupture

IFIRST SAW RYAN through the glass window between the control station and the angiography suite where he was asleep on the procedure table. Fourteen years old, he had presented with a sudden severe headache while at home listening to music in his room and had stumbled into the den holding his head. His parents anxiously drove him to the local hospital, where a hastily done CT scan showed a thin sheen of blood between the frontal lobes of the brain up and down the multiple crevices in the subarachnoid space. This pattern of bleeding on a CT scan typically signals a ruptured intracranial aneurysm, a life-threatening emergency, and is much more common in adults than kids. One-third of those who experience the first hemorrhage, ominously called the sentinel bleed, will die, never having time to make it to the hospital. The aneurysm itself is an area where the blood vessel wall has gradually thinned out until it finally ruptures and blood leaks out under pressure into the space surrounding the brain. Untreated high blood pressure, high cholesterol, cigarette smoking, and being male are all associated with the development of brain aneurysms in adults, but in truth anyone can get one, even kids. In their case the reason is less understood. My adult partners see three or four patients a week with an intracranial aneurysm. In the pediatric world, we may see that in a year.

The tiny vessels that run to and from the brain travel in the subarachnoid space, an anatomical layer typically one millimeter in depth below that plastic wrap–like arachnoid membrane that encases the brain and spinal cord space. If blood is released into it, it collects within it and can irritate the brain, causing severe, send-you-to-the-hospital headaches, seizures, or, if severe enough, death. The next test after the initial CT is usually an angiogram, during which a tiny catheter is snaked through the artery in the groin up into the brain and dye is injected. A continuous series of video X-ray images then show both normal and abnormal blood vessels, and a plan for treatment can be made. All of this is bad and life threatening and very scary if you are a parent or a patient. If you are a neurosurgeon, it means it's time to focus on the task at hand.

My senior partner had been on call during the weekend when Ryan arrived and asked me to assume his care the following morning. I was the newest partner and eager to grow my practice. Hearing that he was initially neurologically intact but with a severe headache, I was reassured that we had time to understand what we were looking at and make a plan for surgery. As we spoke, my partner told me that the interventional radiologist whom I had met once before during my yearlong fellowship was busy at work taking the pictures and videos that I would need to see.

As expected, the angiogram showed an aneurysm where the epicenter of the thin blood clot was. It had two lobes and was around the size of two blueberries. It had formed off the distal anterior cerebral artery on the right, one of the main arteries in the brain, and gave off tiny branches that fed the part of the motor strip responsible for leg movement. The interventional radiologist began to make plans to "coil it"—a method of treatment that occludes the aneurysm from the inside by placing tiny, soft wire fragments into it through the inside of the blood vessels accessed during the angiogram. The tiny wires promote a clot to form within the dome, or outpouching, of the aneurysm while the parent normal vessel stays intact. This internal clot within the dome of the aneurysm itself then reduces the risk of re-rupture. Twenty years ago, at the start of my practice when this occurred, this technique of coiling, which would come to be known as neuro-endovascular surgery, was becoming more popular across the field as more and more neuro-surgeons were learning how to do it. The traditional way of treating a ruptured brain aneurysm is through a craniotomy—by opening the skull—and it can carry a significant chance of morbidity. This field known as neuro-endovascular surgery was new when Ryan presented, but results were quite promising at the time. Indeed over the subsequent years as experience grew, the vast majority of intra-cranial aneurysms would come to be treated in this less invasive manner. It was revolutionary.

But back then, the revolution had yet to occur.

"I am going to embolize it," said the radiologist to the technologists who were assisting him. "Let the family know."

I was surprised and a little taken aback that he had not tried to contact me so that we could discuss the options before forging ahead. I called out from around the windowed partial wall, a little louder and more forceful than I had intended to be, "This patient was handed off to me this morning. Did you talk to anyone already about moving on right to embolization?"

He looked up, surprised to see me.

"Oh, okay," he said in my general direction, mild irritation in his voice at the interruption. "I can get coils in it." He looked up directly at me and asked, "Are you saying that you want to clip it today? Do you have an operating room ready? Because I can treat it right now."

As I think back on this moment nearly two decades ago, the desire to go back in time nearly overwhelms me now.

Yes, I want to have said. *Yes, I am going to clip it later today.* And then after the angiogram was done, I would have spoken to the family, called the OR, and soon afterward, while under the operating microscope, carefully slipped a specially designed titanium spring-loaded clip around the base of the aneurysm, referred to as the neck, effectively excluding the weakened outpouching from the normal circulation and reducing his risk of re-rupture to essentially zero. Just as I had done in training and just as I have done two or three times a year since. Several weeks later, Ryan would have been finishing his physical therapy and back in school.

That memory has no regrets. That memory provides holiday cards and updates on his life that I put in my own cabinet above my desk, like Tim's. His story fades into the others who recovered back to a normal life. His story becomes one that I can let go.

But that is not Ryan's story, and that is not my memory.

"Well, I could," I said hesitantly, "but you seem to think you can coil it?" I only had six weeks as an attending; I could not muster that same degree of assuredness.

"Yep. I'll embolize it now," he said, never looking up. "Let's see what we can get."

Thirty minutes or so later, he had 85 percent of the lesion coiled and no longer showing communication with the normal circulation. There was a portion left untreated just at the takeoff of the vessel, an area that could still rupture again. *I can still see it, despite the nearly two decades that have passed. Right there on the control room screen.*

"I'm not going to coil this last bit. It may clot off the parent vessel." His thought was to avoid a stroke. Simple. Adding another tiny coil could flick off into the parent vessel and clot off, guaranteeing a stroke. The parent vessel of this aneurysm was the anterior cerebral artery on the right side. The blood in that artery goes to nourish the motor and sensory portion of the brain that controls the left leg and foot. If that were to clot off, then he would suffer a stroke in that area and be unable to use that leg. Not a small issue.

"Let's check another angiogram in a few weeks," he said. "My bet is that it will all be clotted off and fine."

NO! It will not be fine! We now know that a partially secured aneurysm with that much left, either by coiling or by clipping, is still risky. I can put a clip all the way across the neck of it this afternoon.

"Sounds good," I say.

The call actually came during my welcome-to-the-practice party. I was on call, a nifty experienced move by my partners.

Our fellow at the time looked directly at me as he took the initial call. Ryan had been home for a week after his two-week stay in the ICU. We managed him through a few issues, and he went home feeling well with pleased parents. Now he was in the emergency room and comatose, his pupils fixed and dilated, a sign of nearly irretrievable brain injury. It was catastrophic. He had re-ruptured the unsecured portion of his aneurysm and he was dying. His parents found him on the floor between his bed and the bathroom, his breath agonal.

The fellow and I drove in together, fast. A senior vascular neuro-surgeon also at the party volunteered to help since it would be hard to clip with all of those coils in it. I was thankful for his presence. Ryan's brain was swollen and the clip difficult to get between the hemispheres. The coils indeed made closing the tips of the aneurysm clip nearly impossible, but my senior vascular partner was able to get my clip to close using a second clip as a bolster. It did not matter. Ryan never woke up, progressing quickly to brain death. It was stunning and swift and terrible. In his last few days, his family had plastered the walls of his ICU room with photographs of Ryan as a younger child, *their beloved child*, as a preteen and athlete. Baseball teams, birthday parties, first bicycle rides, notes and cards from family and friends, all over the walls of the room. Love and warmth and family and faith and friends surrounding him in that hospital bed from all directions.

I have never been able to shake the feeling that Ryan died because I did not speak up when I could have, when I should have. I had failed him. Whether or not the outcome would have been the same,

I would have rather it be because I did what I knew to do, what I was trained to do, instead of leaving his fate to someone else's decision-making. Let me be clear: Now, two decades later, we know so much more about both types of surgery. We know that endovascular surgery is a wonderful option for many patients, and as once hoped, it can reduce the morbidity of surgery drastically. Patients often go home the first day after surgery now, return to work earlier, go back to their lives faster. But we also know now that an aneurysm only partially treated, either open or coiled, is still at risk for rupture.

To this day I have no idea if he would have returned with a re-rupture had I taken him to the OR that same day as the initial angiogram and clipped it. Even now as I write this, the very idea that the same thing would have happened regardless of my actions sounds like a feeble attempt to assuage my guilt. If I had performed the surgery and it had re-ruptured later, I am certain that I would have written an essay similar to this one. Instead of remorse that I did not act, it would have been remorse because I did. People can die. Kids can die. You can do or not do, you can pray or not pray, you can work past the edge of exhaustion, but they still die. Death becomes a part of your daily rhythm. One may become inured to it, but I have yet to find a way to rid myself of it completely. I desperately want it gone, and yet for some odd reason I desperately want to never let it go. Without it, there is no final line to hold. Without it to struggle against, we become less of who we think we are.

My son, Jack, recently moved past the exact age of Ryan when I first met him asleep under the blue sterile drapes in the angiogram suite, so I find myself thinking of him a good bit now. I can see those photos on the walls of his ICU room as Jack poses with his baseball team or stands goofing with his school friends. Sometimes I see those same photos in my closed eyes when I hug Jack or Fair deeply, the way a parent does when they know that soon their child won't tolerate those deep hugs much longer.

The parents were of course devastated when it became time to let him go. There is no place in this time of grief to ask for forgiveness. Forgiveness that would mainly serve only me. Most times the parents want to move past you, want to over time forget the struggle and the intensity of the sadness that you would bring every day as the news became only worse. That lack of resolution is something as pediatric neurosurgeons we often carry with us in some way forever, trying to save the next person just to make up for the failure of the last. Over time, I've come to understand that we make our decisions based on the information we have at the time, that sometimes we act and things are no better, or that we don't act and it's the same. But as I write this, I can still to this very moment see Ryan's aneurysm on the screen, hear those long-ago words spoken from my mouth, and wish to the ends of the earth to know that he forgives me.

On the Morning My Father Died

FOR YEARS, PART of my own family's lore around my father was regarding a particularly important experience during his time in the Mississippi Air National Guard (ANG). He had joined the Air Force Reserve and attended flight school as soon as his college would let him. At each stop in his nonmilitary career, he kept his appointment in the guard and his involvement in flying. By the mid-1980s he had worked his way up to a leadership position in Jackson, Mississippi, flying large C-130 Hercules transport planes. Soon he was offered the ranking position at the ANG base in Meridian with the 186th Tactical Reconnaissance Group. But there were issues there, morale among the most significant. The unit had been allotted F-4 Phantoms, older fighter-bombers from the Vietnam War era. The air force was replacing most of them with the newer F-15 and F-16 so the National Guard units were getting what the air force was phasing out. At least that was the perception at the time.

In addition, this particular group of F-4s had the guns stripped out of their nose cones and reconnaissance cameras put in. The unit had been transformed to a recon unit. Because of this perception of getting the hand-me-downs and the lack of weapons, which took away the fighter pilot persona, morale remained low and issues of unit readiness became the norm.

Into this my father brought his near-limitless optimism and ability to motivate people around him to become better versions of themselves. Early in his tenure there, he had established himself as a talented pilot, having calmly faced the need to dump his fuel tanks and successfully perform a wheels-up landing due to unforeseen hydraulic failure. Over time, he began to effect the turnaround that became a part of this narrative for the remainder of his career and would one day spill over into mine.

His message to the 186th was simple. When called to duty, their pilots were expected to fly into harm's way to get the information to keep as many soldiers on the ground as safe as possible and then fly out. His expectation as their commanding officer was that they were to be the very best pilots in the entire Air National Guard. No longer could they hold on to the idea of falling back on the possibility of shooting their way out of a situation; they had to fly their way out. That's what the best pilots did. Fly like hell.

And that they did. Small successes led to larger ones. No longer would they accept anything less than the fact that they were expected to be the best. Over time the 186th would go on to win top scores in national readiness awards, representing themselves and the military strongly in various missions across the world and achieving prestige among top air force generals and the U.S. Senate itself as the rare Air National Guard unit achieving readiness status equal to that of a full-time U.S. Air Force unit. A decade later, as he approached retirement due to the effects of ALS, my father would be awarded the Mississippi Magnolia Cross for this transformational work at the 186th. Later, on his most honored day, he was awarded the Legion of Merit by the U.S. Air Force, the seventh-highest medal awarded in the military. On the same day celebrating his retirement, my mother pinned a second general's star on his jacket. Then, just like that, his military career—his flying—was done.

What I also know about my father's career as a military pilot is that despite his success and the effect it had on me, it was well more than the triumphs and turnarounds. In his time, he was passed over for promotions and had opportunities move just out of reach for someone who was the son of a dry cleaner from Mississippi. I also remember that despite these disappointments he kept himself positive. He was always grateful for the opportunity to fly, to engage with others around him, to be able to focus his will and energy on something he believed in. It took me some time to get, but perhaps this is the greatest lesson from pilot-father to surgeon-son. To focus less on achievements and recognition and more on connections. Less on noting when the self-perceived limitless trajectory of one's own career inevitably begins to bend its arc toward the horizon and more on how to build up others around you.

Early in my second year of residency, it became clear that my father's ALS had become end stage. I pushed through the final Kübler-Ross stages of grief and went home to spend a week with him as he neared death. Everyone knew why I was there, including him: to say goodbye.

The prior year had been a blur of patients and emergencies and long hours. All of it helping to bury the sadness of his diagnosis and decline. On the two times over the course of the year that I had a week off, I would work at the hospital right up until the last minute. Then Melissa would pick me up at the curb of the hospital entrance, having packed my bags, and we would just barely make the flight. I remember both times I would look down to see that not only was I wearing scrubs on the flight but there was blood on my pants cuff. Just enough for me to see. I think that somehow it made me feel important, as if I were willing to subjugate decorum and even reason for all-consuming work. Early in your training, there is something so powerful about body fluid, sacrificial, that you are willing to be bathed in it. (I remember two of my fellow interns showing up to take the final step of our board exam both covered in bile from a peritoneal tap they had been ordered to perform on a coughing patient with liver failure just an hour before they were to sit for the 8:00 A.M. test.)

A week prior to my arrival, Dad had reluctantly approved a surgically placed feeding tube, all of us persuading him to do it, including me. That was the only procedure that he had agreed to. He had no desire to have a tracheostomy or be put on a ventilator. He knew his death was imminent. He thought the feeding tube would make things easier on everyone else. Unfortunately, he reacted badly to the sedation for it, his blood pressure precipitously dropping during the procedure, and he was admitted to the hospital afterward. This began the slow final decline toward his death. I'm not certain that feeding tube was ever even used.

I had taken an unplanned week off from my neurosurgery residency to be with him, possible only with the death or imminent death of a parent, spouse, or child. For context, there were no weddings or other funerals attended during my residency. Later, I was unable to be a pallbearer for my godmother when she died unexpectedly. I dropped out of sight for friends and extended family for the entire six years. One exception: When my sister-in-law decided to marry in Hawaii in my final year as chief resident, I was initially given permission to fly there on the condition that I return in twenty-four hours. (After negotiation, I was able to stay for seventy-two hours.)

Despite ALS being a disease that primarily affects motor function and not cognition, as his body slowly shut down that week, he was lucid only in stops and starts. Friends would drop by to pay their respects to him and my mother. But as is natural, over time it became my mother, Eve and Sarah, and me with him alone. One last time together as a family.

The morning of my departure, he was lucid, talking to all of us around him. I had my window. I asked everyone else to step out.

I sat next to his bed. I looked down at this once-strong man now lying in the hospital bed, unmoving. I dug the hand nearest me out of the sheets; it was small now, only the tendons and bones showing under the taut skin, the muscles now completely atrophied, the pads underneath the thumb and opposite side of the hand concave. I thought about watching him fly, those hands on the yoke of whatever plane we happened to be in. The hours spent marveling at how they effortlessly passed across the instrument panel, the way he would pull into a turn, or gently set down on a runway in that Aztec, easing to the earth as if he had never left it.

I thought about that stethoscope he had given me years ago, with his own name etched into the bell. The career as a physician, an unrealized dream that I had made a reality for him. Until his diagnosis, he would listen to the stories of patients I had helped to care for, their presenting signs and symptoms, how diagnoses were made, and all the way to recovery or submission. He would have loved the stories to come over the years: the joy of the saves, the grief of the losses, and all the places in between.

Sitting there next to him, I remembered one night he and I were in the car outside my apartment, medical school graduation impending. A new life in Durham immersing myself in residency, hiding away in my work, awaited me. I remember pounding my fists against the steering wheel. *Why am I doing this? How did this become my only option? Why did you set me on this course?* Then the confused anger quickly moving to *Why do you have to be sick? Why now? Why ALS of all things? Why do you have to die now?* Then, finally, *Why am I leaving?*

My father sat silently. The words moved in the air around us. We both quietly began to weep and then embraced for a time. It was the only moment of unabated grief that I saw him fully allow himself. We sat staring forward for a while longer in the car until one of us reached for the door.

Afterward, we walked into my apartment. Melissa was away for the night with her own parents, making plans for future visits to

Durham. Earlier that week, she and I had started an early round of cleaning out in preparation for the move in the next month. The apartment was in chaos because we had begun to thin out clothes and knickknacks to prepare for the sparseness that a five-hundred-square-foot apartment where we would live the first year in North Carolina would afford. I followed him closely while he carefully walked down the hall. I watched as he reached out to use the wall for balance.

I saw him make his way into our bedroom, and I followed him in. The bed had been pulled back from the wall during vacuuming and was still out of place. In the opening between the wall and the bed could clearly be seen the black rubber tubing and metal of the stethoscope that he had given me so long ago. Back in the days when I had considered cardiology as a career, I would lie in bed at night and listen to Mel's heart until we both fell asleep. It must have finally slipped out of my hands one night and fallen out of sight. Then life and my own career choices happened, and the stethoscope lay where it fell long enough to gather a fine layer of dust.

He asked me to pick it up and hand it to him. I watched as he carefully wiped off the dust that had accumulated on it with the handkerchief that he always carried in his pocket, his hands slowly moving around its surfaces. He gently burnished the bell, not an easy task with his hands now so weak, with the weakness always accentuated at the end of the day. His thumb passed over the inscription of his own alternate path—"John C. Wellons, MD"—even our names the same, before he carefully curled it up and placed it in his side jacket pocket, just as the doctor who had given it to him long ago would do.

A NURSE STARTLED me as she came in and out of the room. His unmoving hand was nearly fully enveloped by my own. Sarah checked in and then left just as quickly when she saw me still sitting there as she had left us.

If there was anything redeeming about the whole disease, that balanced out the awfulness of a gradual death, the grief meted out slowly, and the joy stolen from the other times, it was lived out right then in that moment as I formed the words in my head—the last words I would have for my father. I took his atrophied hand in both of mine and looked him in the eyes—at the man who had lived a life I knew only a part of and who had set me on this path. I thought of how profoundly grateful I was to him. He looked up at me and smiled as I spoke. I put his hand to my heart as it nearly beat out of my chest with both grief and gratitude. And love.

ON MY RETURN to work the next day after the late flight back, the current of urgent patient care drew me back in quickly. Life as a new second-year neurosurgery resident was busy and thankfully distracting. There were lives to save and to let go, much easier to focus on them than me.

The next day, I was scheduled to help with an operation on an eleven-year-old with a congenital malformation of the cerebellum and skull base called a Chiari I malformation, named after the man who first described it in the late nineteenth century. This child's particular Chiari blocked the outlet of the fourth ventricle, causing spinal fluid to back up into the center of the spinal cord instead of around it. The symptoms can become quite severe if unheeded. Over the ensuing twenty-five years, this procedure would become a focus of my career and is now the most common operation I do. But I never made it to that child's operation.

Instead of heading to the OR after 6:00 A.M. rounds, I had been told by the chief resident to run up to the neurosurgery ward to handle an issue with a postoperative brain tumor patient. Afterward, instead of turning on a dime and heading down the two flights of stairs to the operating room, I found myself overcome with an exhaustion I had never experienced before. A lack of sleep was nothing new for any of us as neurosurgery residents. It was not uncommon for us to be up two nights in a row in those days and still operate on the morning of the third day.

But this was different. Just forty-eight hours before, I had been at my father's bedside. On my return, I had immediately begun the ongoing long shift.

I quickly stepped into the empty break room just behind the nurses' station. At that moment I didn't have the capacity to care about where I was supposed to be or what anyone else thought I should be doing. I just sat down in a chair in front of a computer with its blinking cursor, put my head in my arms on the counter, and was instantly lost to sleep.

When you are profoundly tired, you quickly enter a cycle of REM sleep, during which your eyes dart around under your closed lids and you dream. I was there within seconds.

I dreamed that I was walking with my father, just the two of us together. We were in our backyard at home in southern Mississippi around the tall magnolia tree I would climb as a child. He paused to sit in one of those 1970s-style plastic-lattice folding chairs that were always in that backyard. I reached up to take a branch while he watched me. Then another and another until I was high up in that tree, higher up than I ever remember being in real life.

All of a sudden there was a piercing noise. It was high-pitched and all around me.

I looked down from the upper branches of the tree. My father had no reaction. It seemed that only I could hear it.

I held on with my elbows wrapped around the branches, my hands on my ears, the sound was so loud. I wanted it to stop. It had to stop.

"Make it STOP!" I yelled out loud.

I woke up and sat straight up in the chair.

The sound was my pager, sitting right next to the computer where I had put it before I laid my head down.

In those disorienting initial seconds after waking up, still exhausted, I thought of only the very present. *What's happening? Someone is coding. I'm needed in the ER. Damn it, I am supposed to be in the OR right now.*

I looked down at the number on my pager screen, wincing, confused, trying to make coherent sense of its information. *What had I slept through? What the hell was I thinking?*

The area code was 601, which takes in all of southern Mississippi, then a series of unrecognizable numbers. *What the . . . ?* The three numbers 911 were tacked on at the end, a signal from my family.

Then in the next few seconds, I had a series of painful realizations as I quickly put the jumbled pieces together, living them all in an instant: *my father's ALS, his decline, that final week, his intermittent lucidity, our goodbye.* I had no protection from it all.

And now, I knew, *his death.*

IN THE TWENTY-FIVE years since that morning, the rawness of that moment has never left me. Somehow it was simultaneously two very different things, a long, drawn-out dying in which suffering took its toll on him and us. Death, then, welcome when it finally came, was also a rapid shock, a moment of realized grief that was deep and stunning and still felt now.

On occasion I have seen that same grief in the faces of the parents and loved ones of the children I am taking care of after something terrible and ultimate has happened to their child and there is no return from it. But this was my first true loss, my first true grief. For a while, with each patient who died despite our best efforts, I would relive this feeling. I think it was the avoidance of this profound grief that pushed me so hard in my early years. Loss is endemic to neurosurgery; there was no way to get around that then or now. But witnessing the grief over and over again did in time enable me to understand that grief is as much a part of this life as joy. Indeed, the ultimate grief of loss is heightened by the intense joy that love brings. Love for the one forever lost. Without one, the other is muted, less real. One must coexist with the other.

In dreams in the years since his death, my father and I have walked together around the base of that same magnolia tree and flown together in the Aztec in and among the clouds. It's in those places that he hears those stories of my patients that have come in some way to be my stories too. We've sat in those 1970s plastic-lattice backyard chairs to watch my own children, whom he never met in life, play and romp and walk out to the far garden in the same backyard that I grew up in. In this way, he's witnessed the births and baptisms and moments of grace and joy with them that his early dying took away, his words to me in those dreams never again goodbye.

That photograph referred to in "Ninety Minutes from You by Ground" that I keep on my desk is of him standing next to his F-4 Phantom. Wearing that olive-drab flight suit, his helmet and flight bag under his arm, he is casually leaning on the narrow antenna coming straight off the nose cone of the plane, parallel to the ground. On his face a huge smile, larger than I typically remember, caught more in a mid-laugh. Pushed back on the base of the antenna is a wooden propeller, taken from who knows where. It takes a second to realize that a wooden propeller is not supposed to be on the nose cone of this high-speed jet aircraft. I remember when Dad and I first found this photograph together, in his desk drawer at our family home. His hands just starting to weaken from his ALS. With his guidance I separated our findings into various piles. He told me how his chief flight mechanic had slid that propeller down the antenna of the nose cone. Then, waiting for him on the flight line, he had told my father that he had finally figured out how to make the colonel's damn plane go faster, so would he now please stop asking him. Then, as they both laughed, he had snapped the photograph of my father, the commander of the Magnolia Militia, as they all called themselves, standing next to his beloved F-4 Phantom. Neither of them ever knowing that the lasting image of that shared moment would one day sit on the desk of the colonel's son, that very photograph one of the few links to his father's storied and heralded past, both pulling him back and pushing him forward.

17

Birth

*T*HERE'S NOT SUPPOSED *to be a baby at this point.*
An infant had just appeared above the sterile drapes of the operative field, sprawled on its tiny doll-like back and carefully cradled in two gloved hands. The newborn's skin was a dusky and pale blue, mottled all over. Seconds ago, it had been a twenty-six-week fetus we were operating on inside the womb to repair a myelomeningocele. Then there was a flash of blood, and suddenly a tiny child, a girl, was there with us.

The placenta had emergently pulled away from the uterine wall. Instead of a lifeline, sharing blood with the fetus, it began to rapidly syphon that, and the baby's life, away. Three months earlier than normal, the *entire third trimester* gone.

As the umbilical cord was quickly clamped and cut, I watched the baby's chest. Not even the faintest shudder of effort. Stillness amid the growing chaos around her. Looked at again, it could have easily been a part of a lung or liver or some other organ newly excised rather than this new being freshly pulled into the world.

The gloved hands shifted. A single ghostly white limb unfurled to dangle limply below its tiny body.

Then, just as quickly as it appeared, the baby was gone, thrust into a pair of outstretched arms and taken off the surgical field draped in a blanket. A crowd of neonatologists had formed behind me and turned away the moment they received the child.

The sound in the room rushed back in. Multiple alarms. Urgent voices all at once, from all directions.

"We need to open the trauma blood!"

"I need a syringe of epi now."

"Careful, careful. Get her right here in the warmer . . ."

"Suck here. I can't see what's bleeding!"

A small tray of instruments was bumped off a side table and crashed to the ground. The door to the OR banged open as a second crash cart was brought in. The neonatologists slid the baby into the warming bay, blankets opened up now to the radiant heat from the warmers designed for this very reason. Soon the infant disappeared behind a wall of shoulders.

I turned back to see the placenta trace a low arc in the air, slung back in haste by one of the maternal-fetal surgeons into a blue plastic basin held up by the scrub nurse. I watched as she carefully folded its edges into the basin and handed it off to more outstretched arms. It too disappeared into the crowd. I remembered from the last delivery I was a part of—*thirty years ago as a medical student*—that someone in the growing sea of people in the OR would try to draw blood off it for testing. *No, no, that's not right. The last delivery I remember was Fair, my own daughter, now thirteen. I remember her calm face. There was no cry at her beginning, only soft breathing. And joy. So much joy.*

Back below me, waves of blood heaved out of the mother's open uterus. This was beyond anything we dealt with in neurosurgery. The blood loss here was *audible,* a low rush below us. The two maternal-fetal surgeons furiously worked to find the source and control it. Blood soaked the surgical drapes down onto the floor. The two of them, gowns bloodstained up to their mid-forearms now, calling out for sutures and large instruments with unfamiliar names. I heard a split-second decision made to attempt to save the uterus in this young mother. *What decision would my own wife want? Way back, before we had our own children. On our own five-year journey of IVF cycle after cycle to our own family.*

Anesthesia had the IV lines "wide open" to rapidly infuse fluid to replace the lost volume and push medicines designed to bring the blood pressure back up. The mother had moved deeper into hemorrhagic shock. Large plunger-shaped syringes were connected to plump red bags and the blood contained in them pulled out of the bag and pushed into the mom emergently in two motions. Draw out. Push in. Draw out. Push in. After a few cycles, the blood pressure stopped its precipitous drop and began to stabilize. *All the medicine in the world can do only so much,* I remember someone telling me in a long-ago ER trauma bay. *The best treatment for blood loss is blood gain.* My own scrub pants back then covered with blood. I remember turning my face away, my fists clenched with the realization of failure. That failure, long ago, meant death in the ED. My introduction.

I looked back again as the neonatology team had successfully intubated the infant and kick-started the first few breaths with a tiny oxygen bag and mask, each forced breath barely a twitch of the respiratory therapist's fingers on the bag, the tiny lungs so fragile. One bag full of air pushed in too rapidly, too uncontrolled, and the baby's lungs would rupture, an unrecoverable deadly injury caused by the very person trying to save her.

Two fronts now raged around me. As two battles against death had appeared in the moments after everything had turned, I realized that I was standing there still holding my tiny micro-instruments in the air. Utterly useless. In an instant, I had become only a spectator.

The whole reason we were there was to repair the open spinal cord. Fetal surgery for spina bifida can make a tremendous difference in a child's function later in life. I didn't really believe it before I took this job nearly a decade ago. My own heuristics formed in the decade before coming here had held the day. I wanted proof. Proof beyond the scientific papers. I wanted to see the results myself. To hear their *stories*.

Now I am an integral part of that team. Noel, who had given his career over to fetal neurosurgery, died too early in life, and in place of him, I am the one who gives the national talks and publishes the papers and travels across borders to help start programs. The big shot. Right. *Okay, lean in here. Listen up, folks. When everything goes to hell, make sure as the pediatric neurosurgeon you stand there frozen.*

My gloves are now sticky, gummy, as the blood dries while I turn back and forth from team to team. The sudden spectator. Somehow now alone in a spasm of chaos and voices and blood.

I watch as Kelly, now fully in her role as lead maternal fetal surgeon, places thick chromic sutures in the uterine wall to stop the bleeding while the other surgeon holds the uterus tight, squeezing down with all his might to help stanch the flow.

Minutes before, the room had been quiet, focused on the monitor where I worked to repair the defect. My assistant was a sixth-year neurosurgery resident and destined for a career in pediatric neurosurgery. She had recently committed to an extra year of training tacked on to the end of an already long seven years. The wall-mounted video monitor showed the tips of our instruments working in unison. This was not going smoothly. Last week, it was her hands sewing up the back as I pulled each stitch just tight enough to hold. But not today. Today it was back to her assisting me. From the time of anesthesia induction on, each step in this particular case had been challenging, pushing back in some way.

Mom and Dad had been told of the risks. There is no way to pull the punches when consenting to this surgery. The mother's life is at risk. If something were to go wrong, we would fight first to save her, then the fetus. She was a cosmetologist and he an IT technician, with two other children together. Funds had been raised through a GoFundMe account so that they could afford to take the time away from work to stay close by once their daughter was released from the hospital after surgery. Christmas for the two other kids would take a backseat this year, and the kids understood why. *Sister needed surgery.* They were all already sacrificing for this little girl yet to be in this world. No hesitation.

At every check-in step the day of surgery from 5:00 A.M. on, they were courteous, engaged, invested, and fully convinced that closing the defect was the best decision and that all the sacrifices were worth the risk. *Just look at all this kindness surrounding us.*

After looking for a suitable entry corridor through the uterine wall with an ultrasound, Kelly had carefully opened and widened the hole with sutures and a stapler that helped to avoid robust bleeding from the highly vascular uterine wall edges. The ultrasound confirmed what we saw beneath us: The fetus was rotated away, the back and operative site hidden from view. Typically, this would not be an issue, but this time the fetus did not move around inside the uterus smoothly as we tried to roll it over. The standard movements done to bring the fetus back up into view weren't working. The surgical site on the fetal back kept falling right back to where it was before, away from where I could reach it.

I see it happening again now. Someone finally gets two fingers underneath the right side of the uterus. Using the forceps, I carefully take hold of the healthier parts of the fetal skin and rotate the fetus in the womb up to me.

The dome of the undeveloped spinal cord bulges up through the open uterus wall. The neural tissue is there on the surface, more diffuse and less defined than normal. *Has anything about this case been normal at this point?* The rest of the spinal cord trails off underneath it, disappearing into the spinal canal. That I can see clearly. Our usual goal is to cut around the exposed part, separating the neural tissue—the placode—from the skin in order to let it settle down into the canal. Then we would either dissect out a layer of dura to sew over it or, if the tissue is too wet-tissue-paper-like, put a tiny little tissue graft in place. After that, we would carefully create a surgical plane—a space—between the back muscles and the skin all the way out to the sides of the fetus, past the visible edges of the uterine opening, in order to free up the skin just enough to stretch it across the midline and close the defect. It is the rare blind dissection in our field.

None of that plan would play out today. Mom's blood pressure had been up and down since nearly the beginning, the monitors intermittently alarming. The anesthesia team excitedly gave various intravenous medicines to adjust her pressure while the pediatric cardiologist in the corner of the room watched the image of the fetal heart on the monitor and called out as issues with the fetal blood flow came and went.

Finally, I'd opened the bubble of fluid to let off pressure and had started to cut around the flat placode to separate it away from the normal skin.

Alarms came from over the drapes from the anesthesia monitors. A calm voice said, "We have a blood pressure spike. We're treating it."

From the cardiologist monitoring the fetal heart: "We've got a filling defect showing here." A sign of early blood loss, from somewhere.

The placode again rolled away from me. *Damn it. This may not be doable.* Kelly and I tried to rotate it back up together. Gently pushing from below and ever so slightly pulling from above.

In a flash, there was a wall of blood that washed over my fingers, from the knuckles down. A tsunami of blood overtook my field of vision in my surgical loupes and filled up the entire uterus within seconds.

"Abruption!" Kelly called out urgently, signaling that the placenta had begun to acutely pull away from the inside of the uterus.

Our team had been doing these operations together for a decade, and this had never happened. In a flash, we were fully in the middle of it. Everything was at risk here. The unborn child could die. The mother could die. Both could die. There was nothing else in the entire universe to those of us in that room except for that fetus and that brave mother.

I'm holding my tiny forceps and tiny scissors and blood has welled up to my wrists. Somewhere in there I still have a hold of the flimsy back skin of the fetus.

"We're delivering this baby," said Kelly matter-of-factly. "Jay, you have to let go."

Let go.

I have never been at this place before. Where I must step away. When the monitors alarm and the blood is pooling and things are turning upside down. It has been drilled in me to step forward, not back. Now I am indeed frozen, ineffectual. In the way.

"Let go, Jay."

In one motion, I release the fetus and bring my hands back. Kelly and her team step into the gap. With one deft flash of steel, the opening in the uterus is extended and she reaches inside.

THE BLEEDING HAS been stopped, the mom and now newborn stable. Kelly has walked out to speak with the father. The remaining maternal-fetal surgeon and his assistant are methodically closing up the abdomen. The atmosphere on the other side of the drapes among the anesthesia team is much calmer. No alarms, no pushing blood, no furious chatter. I hear a low nervous chuckle in response to something said.

I look over to the Isolette, where the breathing tube down the infant's windpipe is helping to bring needed oxygen into the lungs. Gently the chest rises up and down. The nurse carefully squirts a microdosed medicine down that tube, the veins too small for IVs. The heart rate is fast, but everyone over there is calm about it. I see smiles at the edges of their masks. Someone leans casually against the wall. I assume all is normal. At least normal for whatever this is.

I realize in a flash that I still need to close the back.

Still our scrub nurse for all the fetal cases, Melissa sees me look-ing and says to me from across the room, "I have your other instru-ments sterile and ready."

I lean into the crew gathered around the baby, my sterile gown now long contaminated, and tell them that I would like to close the back before the baby leaves the room. *I want to finish what I started.* I am on task now.

"Can you do it in fifteen minutes?" the lead neonatologist asks. "We're stable now, but it sure would be nice to be in a unit by then."

I nod and head back out to rescrub. Without asking, my senior resident quietly comes with me to do the same. In the same way that I need her help in this, I know her well enough to know that she needs to help. To be a part of what we know how to do. Closure. Of the baby's back. Of our roles as neurosurgeons. Of one of our last fetal cases together before she rotates back onto the adult service for her last year, then ultimately away the next for a fellowship.

We enter together. We are silent at the scrub sink. Melissa hands us our towels. Then our gowns and gloves and we are ready.

I instinctively move toward the mother, to the place where I had been when all of this happened. Then I realize my lapse and turn toward the Isolette. The neonatal team clears a path and we begin.

Soon, our hands are moving together in the closure. We carefully separate out each layer and bring them together with tiny sutures. The final few hold in the now-pinkening skin, puckering slightly, and we are done.

In one final and fitting reminder, no one can find a dressing small enough for the back of a twenty-six-week-old baby. *I've never needed one before in this OR.*

Kelly comes back in the room after several minutes talking to the husband.

"First thing I told him was that there was a placental abruption and that we had to deliver the baby. Then that both Mom and his little girl were stable," she said to the room. "All things considered, he was okay after he recovered from the shock of the news."

She turned to me alone and asked, "What do you think his first question to me was?"

I was quiet. The resident intently applied a makeshift dressing to the baby's back that she had cut down from a larger dressing.

And I somehow knew what she was going to say, and as she did, I thought of that wave of blood and those alarms. That very feeling that washed over me at the same time when I realized I would need to step away. How this took every bit of each one of the people in this room to pull this off, our team of nearly a decade, to bring Mom and baby back.

Let go, Jay.

"Did you hear me, Jay?" Kelly asked.

Let go.

"His first question to me was if you got her back closed."

—·•·—

18

A Mississippi Nick

THE SON OF a bitch chopped me with an ax!"

A man had just burst through the doors into the ED clutching a rag to the front of his neck, it and all of his clothes soaked in sticky wet blood. He looked to be around thirty, was ghostly white and heavyset in the way former high school football linemen become over the years. As he stood wild-eyed just inside the door, the blood spilled up around his fingers, ran down his arm, and pooled on the floor. Behind him, the automatic doors, caught between fully open and closed, spasmed in their frames. A car sped off into the darkness.

"Get him to Trauma 4, stat!" a voice rang out.

I was diverted by the charge nurse from my current job of taking a tray of urine samples to the lab and pushed into the trauma bay, temporarily delaying the fate of five people with potentially positive drug screens, bladder infections, or pregnancies. The man lay sprawled across a gurney; bloody footprints traced his steps across the room.

"Get over here," said a nurse, trying to hold him down. "He's going to bleed out."

As a fourth-year student in the spring of my last year in medical school, I had signed on to do the emergency medicine rotation for two main reasons. The first was an opportunity to hone my sewing skills in the "Suture Box," a windowless room on the back hall of the emergency department where fourth-year students would close up any minor lacerations that presented during their shift. The "Box" was a room that had all types of sutures in colorful boxes lining the shelves, and all shapes of needles, sizes of sutures, really anything you could think of. If you needed to close a complicated stellate eyebrow laceration, there was tiny 6-0 Prolene monofilament. Just next to that was an eye-level sign bolted to the wall that read, "Rule #4: DO NOT SHAVE THE EYEBROWS." There were no other bolted-down rules. Only this particular one appeared at the time to have survived the evolutionary cull. There was broad, strong 1-0 Vicryl for sewing up under the skin across a joint where there would be near-constant shear forces working to pull the wound apart. (For some mysterious reason, the suture 0-0 number goes up the smaller the suture gets.) Tattered books, highlighted and dog-eared, lined the lowest shelf for quick reference. Many a burgeoning Mississippi surgeon had spent weekend nights there as a fourth-year medical student.

The second reason to be there was the shift-based schedule and favorable hours. After three years and nine months of early week-end mornings in the anatomy lab, late nights rounding with the resident-run services, and basically spending every waking hour convincing any surgeon in visual range that I was the hardest-working medical student since Harvey Cushing himself—the founder of neurosurgery—in order to match into the competitive field of neurosurgery, I was ready to cruise just a little. It was often said that the best time of your neurosurgery residency was between when, midway through your fourth year of medical school, you learned you had matched into an actual residency position and when you actually started it in the ensuing July.

The Ax Man, as he quickly became known, had quieted down, and the dirty saturated rag was quickly replaced with cleaner gauze, the moment of the switch marked by a single spurt of bright red blood nearly hitting the swivel lights above.

"Well, that ain't too good," a voice drawled from behind me.

Hamp Frye, the trauma chief resident, walked past me and to the foot of the bed, the position of control of the room. Hamp was pure Mississippi Delta through and through, never rattled, always calm. Occasionally, it seemed, near comatose. I knew folks like him from my college years. I hunted duck with them in the fields around Greenwood and drank beer with them in the same fields at night, dancing with their girlfriends' friends while the towering campfire sent sparks up to blend with the starry sky. I pictured Hamp growing up the same way. I could see him warming his hands on the camp stove inside a duck blind in Tchula, likely swigging a little bourbon to keep warm in the frigid Delta morning.

His team of white-coated and scrub-wearing surgery residents were sprawled across three other acute rooms, sorting through a gunshot wound to the abdomen and a teenager with a fractured pelvis from a car accident. Hamp stood with me alone. The persistent beep of the Ax Man's pulse oxygenation monitor showed an elevated heart rate from blood loss and agitation, but normal oxygenation. The sedative the nurse gave him when we were wrestling him to the bed had started to kick in. The pressure I held on his neck had stopped the bleeding for the moment.

"I estimate there's about four layers of closure there, Wellons. Let me give you a hand." We prepped the skin around the wound, holding one gloved finger on the main pumper that shot up a geyser of blood each time I shifted my finger in order to clean the wound itself with sterile Betadine.

"That's the carotid."

"What the hell's the cartodid?" the man yelled out as we laid sterile towels out around the wound. "SON OF A BITCH! That hurts!" he called out as he reached up to pull the towels away from his neck.

Hamp quickly grabbed the man's hand, looked him in the eye, and said, all traces of laconic southern boy gone from his voice, "*Sir, you have a cut in the main blood vessel that goes to your brain. If* we don't sew this up now, you will die. DIE. DEAD. Do you understand? Now hold still!"

Silence. Stillness.

Hamp reached down with a needle driver poised over the wound, my finger on the carotid. I could feel it bounding beneath my finger, the blood pushing up to his brain past where I had compressed it just enough. Too much and the brain could be starved of crucial oxygen-containing blood.

"On the count of three, you pick up your finger, then put it back down like I'm a kid and you are helping me tie my shoes and don't want me to lose the tightness of the knot. Understood?"

"Yes, sir," I responded.

"One . . . two," he counted. "Three!"

At three I lifted my finger up just as Hamp's needle driver flashed down past me. The sharp edges of the hole were visible because the blood pulsed up in a series of single powerful bright red columns that shot up and over the edge of the bed. I would never forget the power of a single human heartbeat after that and would reference that very moment when teaching residents and students over the years. After the first figure-of-eight stitch, I quickly put my finger back down on the suture now loosely covering the hole. He tied the knot, being careful to cinch it down without ripping it out of the wall of the vessel. I picked up my finger again, nothing. No spurting. All that was visible was the pulsing of the exposed carotid and the sharp edges of filleted open muscle. I reached over to cut the suture tails of his knot. Once the carotid bleeding had stopped, we could get a better chance of assessing the overall wound, a fairly clean slice. It looked as if it cleaved the muscle above the carotid sheath in two and just nicked the carotid. Any deeper and he would have likely bled out in the car ride to the ED.

The ED attending came in quickly, followed by the charge nurse.

"Just what in the hell is happening here, Frye? Where's the chart?

Are you doing a procedure without notifying the ED attending? I'm not even sure if we have a name!"

Stripping off his gloves, Hamp looked up at the two of them glaring at him. His body relaxed. The Delta boy came back out again.

"Hey, Doc, no problem here, just a little Mississippi nick. I'm just helping Watson here get a little sewing done," he said, purposely mangling my name. "I'm headed back up to the OR now for that hot appy you all found for us." As he said this, he smiled and started to back out of the room.

Just as he disappeared, he said, "Now make sure you wash that out a little with some clean saline before you close, Watson." Then he was gone.

The ED attending looked at the nurse, then at me, then the prepped-out slash in the neck, and walked out.

I irrigated the wound with a liter of sterile saline fluid in the trauma bay, then rolled the Ax Man back to the Box. He stayed under the drapes the whole time. When we wheeled in and stopped, he spoke again.

"Can I talk yet?"

"Yep," I said. "I'm going to put some numbing medicine all the way around this thing so I can sew you up. This is going to take a while."

After numbing him up, I began the long process of repairing the two severed edges of the sternocleidomastoid muscle, important for turning the head. Repairing muscle is not easy, particularly really big muscles that move the neck around. A standard series of interrupted sutures placed in the muscle just slide out along the parallel muscle fibers. Luckily there was a chapter on what to do in one of the books on the shelves. I laid the open book out on the counter behind me for reference as I worked, repeating a ritual I was sure had been done time and time again in that very room over the years.

"Is it bad, Doc?" he asked.

I told him it was getting better, that he would live, which all things considered was me trying to set the bar really low for the final results of the neck closure. As I worked, he told me about his cousin who was his best friend. That he had made the mistake of asking out his cousin's girlfriend. That's what caused the fight. That and some cheap whiskey. His cousin had confronted him, and the two of them had traded punches in the house, the yard, and the tool-shed. Finally, he had his cousin pinned and was pummeling him in the face to try to end it. That's when his cousin reached out blindly, got his hand on the short ax propped up against the wall in the tool-shed, and took his swing.

"It's not like I was punching him that hard, Doc," he said from under the blue drapes.

On and off after the story I would have to remind him not to sing as I worked, since the movement made the stitching harder and frankly I did not need it to be harder at this point in my career.

When I was finally done closing the whole wound, there was no one available to tell me if it looked okay. He now had a pretty good resemblance of an intact neck, at least I thought so. It looked like the pictures in the book. I carefully bandaged it and gave him instructions on how to clean the wound, starting in a few days. Within a few minutes, I heard a ruckus in the hall.

"He's my family!" a voice said loudly. "My cousin! I'M GOING IN THERE!"

Seconds later, a man even larger than the patient but clearly, as we say in Mississippi, blood kin ran into the room. His face was bruised and swollen to the point of both eyes being nearly completely shut. What I could see in his eyes, though, was fear. Fear of what he would find here in the back room of the emergency department. Fear followed by remorse that I imagine set in quickly as the rage and anger abated. I was certain it must have been his tire squeals that I heard at the ED door because the Ax Man had said that no one else was around when his cousin had confronted him.

He scanned the room and quickly settled on his cousin now sitting up on a stretcher, drapes crumpled on the floor, his clothes stained deeply red.

"Damn, Red!" he said. "What happened to you?"

The Ax Man, now known as Red, looked right at his cousin. Eyes hot. Forearm muscles tight. Several moments passed. I tensed, moving the suture tray with its sharp objects off to the side, waiting to hear his next comment. I gripped down on a hemostat as if I could somehow defend myself with it if things went south.

Then, after a moment longer: "Damn bar fight, that's all. Some drunk jerk with a broken bottle. What you doin' here?"

And that was it. The anger of the attempted jilt, the fight spilling out into the yard, the swing of the ax, the screech of the car driving off, all of it disappeared. Right in that very moment, the narrative changed forever. In no version of the story told later will Red have struck blow after blow long after he should have stopped or been slashed in a wild blow by his drunken, jealous cousin. As I listened to the two of them talk, Red on the gurney, his cousin standing right next to him, I could hear the story morphing into one in which his cousin came to his aid after a vicious attack by a drunken assailant at a bar, the two of them fighting side by side until the bottle slash that led to a wild ride to the hospital. Their kinship, their friendship, saved forever.

I realized I still held the hemostat in my hand at the ready and relaxed, letting it fall into the tray with a clatter. Red hopped off the gurney and draped his arm over his cousin's shoulder. They both turned to leave, laughing loudly at the blood on his pants. I walked toward the exit with them, toward those same automatic doors that Red had presented to earlier that night, trying to give them a prescription for antibiotics for the wound, more gauze for dressing changes. Red just shook his head as the two of them walked out into the night.

"All good, Doc," said Red the Ax Man over his shoulder. "My cousin here will take good care of me."

———·———

19

Luke's Jump

O<small>N THE THIRD</small> jump of the race, things went to hell. The dusty cloud of tumbling riders and dirt bikes finally came to a stop right in front of the trackside bleachers packed with eager and suddenly horrified parents. Giant floodlights, dotted by swarming insects in the warm fall evening, turned the late dusk into day, spotlighting the chaotic scene in front of them. Slowly, one by one, the riders sat up, rubbed their heads, and waved to the crowd. Parents pulled up, mid-run down to the gate that opened onto the track, relieved. Tentative laughter spread across the crowd, a few early claps.

One boy, however, did not rise, still on the track, his crumpled form unmoving. A spreading pool of blood began to form under his head. Silence set back in. *Whose boy is that? Is that Luke?* That boy in the dust was indeed Luke, Luke Nolan, and he would not sit up again for quite some time.

With his father watching from the trackside bleachers, Luke, then twelve years old, had accelerated up the dirt hill after gaining speed on a quick straightaway during his first, and only, time around the track, just as the riders around him were doing. Then, somehow, someone's wheel caught another and the chaos began. On the first bounce back to earth, Luke was thrown off the bike, and his strapped-on helmet somehow flew off his head. With the second bounce, the handlebar of one of the tumbling motorcycles pierced his skull and gouged out a one-inch-deep rough trough in the skull and brain along the left side, his dominant hemisphere, where the areas of the brain that regulate language and speech are represented. More often than not, this is a non-survivable injury. The patient dies at the scene.

Luke's father, pushing to his son's side through the gathering crowd, reflexively lifted the boy off the dirt track and swept him into someone's vehicle for a fast ride to the local hospital. Whether the right thing would have been to wait for an ambulance will never be known. Astonishingly, he had no spine injury, the most common reason for on-scene immobilization. After a quick head wrap by the emergency personnel at the hospital, done to hold pressure and stanch the bleeding, the boy had been emergently sent to us via ambulance. The page went out in the early evening notifying relevant teams of his impending arrival. We were there as the ambulance emptied him into the trauma bay. His father stepped out of the ambulance and walked briskly alongside the gurney.

I had come down to the ED despite my resident's presence there because I had just finished an afternoon case lasting well into the evening and had yet to retrieve my backpack for my bike ride home. Still in my first year of practice, I was eager to be involved from the very beginning, perhaps some of my residency staying with me then. Melissa was a junior medical resident and destined to be chief medicine resident some years later. Her call was equally busy managing nonsurgical issues and she was often in the hospital overnight. There was no cozy dinner or interesting conversation beckoning me from home. I felt the familiar rush of adrenaline setting in as I walked through the ED. After I peeked under the hastily applied but lifesaving head wrap, I quickly realized that I would not be heading home for the next several hours and shifted gears.

Once I had glanced over the CT scan of the boy's head showing immense damage to the skull and underlying brain, I brought the father into the emergency department consultation room to discuss the impending surgery. I also needed to obtain consent. The absence of consent to do the surgery when there is a parent present could be construed as battery, as odd as that sounds. So, consent is therefore critical to proceed. (If there is no parent or relative available, then consent can be deemed emergent and two attending physicians are necessary to approve it.) Back in the days of residency, this conversation was way more about the consent than the connection. That would change for me forever on this night as well.

I was standing for the conversation, as was the father, our eyes at the same height. He wore a goatee, his beard mostly unshaven around it. His thin blue jean jacket was faded and his baseball hat dusty, dark hair underneath matted with sweat. His eyes were red, his face creased; concern and the effects of sustained intensity began to set in. We found ourselves alone in the room. The light box held select films on it showing the devastation to the boy's skull, the bluish light casting across us both. I introduced myself by name as the pediatric neurosurgeon on call. As I did, his chin dropped to his chest. His hand came up to cover his eyes. It was early in my career. I want to say that I reached out and put a hand on his shoulder to comfort him. Even quickly, with the need to get to the OR paramount. That's what I would do now. It's what 95 percent of the pediatric neurosurgeons that I know would do now. Strike the balance. Compassion and focus. Then on to the work. But I was yet to experience the hundreds of moments like this to come. I didn't have those lessons yet. *Get the consent,* I told myself. *Just get to the OR.*

So instead, I looked down to give him a moment to get his composure and mumbled out how hard I knew this must be. There is no perfect space for this. Inside the room is too chaotic, the parent distracted by the child critically ill next to them, the movement of the nurses and doctors around nearly too much for any parent to bear. Just outside the door of the room is an issue because other patients can hear, a practice no longer tolerated by privacy laws.

The final face-to-face option is in a consultation room, often plainly decorated with three to four chairs, a table with a box of tissues, and a single piece of muted art on the wall. These days, a computer to display images has replaced the light box, which has gone the way of pagers and handwritten notes.

As I looked down—distracted as I thought about needing to call the OR board to get the team mobilized, making sure the right labs were drawn, remembering to call the PICU to notify them that this patient would need an ICU bed postoperatively, as well as twenty-three other things that needed to take place in order for this to move forward, *We also need to cross match blood*—I noticed the father's shoes. There, slightly higher, on the cuff of his blue jeans and spilling down onto his socks, I could make out a vaguely familiar grayish color amid blood that had made its way onto his clothes. It was brain matter. His own son's brain matter. Mixed with blood and hair and dirt and grass, right there on his person, the blood and muck creating a dark red sheen on his shirt, the front of his pants, and onto the cuff. In a flash I could picture him stooping down on that dusty track, lifting him up, doing the only thing he knew how, to act. To get his son to care. I looked up at the father right then and felt just a splinter of the horror of what he must have been feeling, the unimaginable pain. Then we locked eyes. He told me the boy's name and choked out that they loved racing motorcycles together. Within minutes I was in the operating room trying to save his son, but the image of that father standing there crying, part of his son's brains down on his own pants leg, remained with me as I operated.

Pediatric neurosurgery tends to be more urgent than other fields, even within the broader field of neurosurgery. At the two places I have worked as faculty, we didn't even know about more than a third of the operations just forty-eight hours before they happened. Conversely, just forty-eight hours before we met on an operating table, these patients were not patients at all, they were people living their lives and thinking their thoughts, blithely unaware that anything was wrong. I'm not sure that I was keyed into this fact as a medical student or neurosurgery resident. It did seem that everything we did back then, adult or pediatric, was an emergency. And far more of our time as trainees outside the actual operating room was spent in the emergency department or intensive care units taking care of critically ill people rather than the more structured and sedate outpatient clinic where other specialties dwell.

But we were young and drawn into an intense field. Urgent was adrenaline. Urgent was an opportunity to operate. Urgent was a story to tell each other on the rare day off. It was only later, when I became an attending, and then a parent, that urgent took on a different meaning. Turns out urgent was someone's child. Urgent was someone's whole world, dependent on the decision you were about to make. Recently, I sat across the table from a middle-aged Muslim woman in the cramped family discussion room of the PICU, moments after I had given her the diagnosis of a brain tumor in her only child.

"Take care of him, Doctor, I beg you," she said, the edges of her hijab wet with tears. "He is my sun and my moon and every single star in my sky."

Over time I came to realize that these urgent cases are what I call the public health mission of pediatric neurosurgery. At the very core of what we should be doing as a field is ensuring that the needs of the community we belong to are taken care of. Within this model, a parent should be able to expect that their child will have the care they need if they need it, be it for a new diagnosis of juvenile diabetes requiring access to a pediatric endocrinologist, a broken arm necessitating pediatric orthopedic care, or a brain, spine, or spinal cord injury or issue requiring surgery. Our role as pediatric neurosurgeons is to take care of those who need assessment and specialized care, and often to go to the operating room emergently for things like trauma, blood clots in the brain, or herniation from hydrocephalus, to name a few. Less emergent but still urgent are things that need to be added on the schedule to get taken care of in the next day or so. These fit somewhere in highly complex and mysteriously "leveled" OR board classification schemes that determine case order across North America and the world. This latter group includes things like spina bifida, pediatric brain tumors, and a host of other things that generally go bad if not sorted out in a day or two. As we progress in our careers, I would argue that our role progresses from putting our heads down and being a part of this process to later helping set up a better system to make sure it is happening and happening well. The lucky among us get to be a part of both of those.

I operated on Luke multiple times. With the dirt from the track came all types of microorganisms. Infection set in, but with aggressive washout operations, excellent infectious disease specialists, and strong antibiotics, we were able to clear him. The initial surgery that first night was to clean out bits of racetrack and grass from the damaged brain, remove the fractured and contaminated skull fragments, and control the bleeding from the torn skin. Fortunately, there was enough skin left to be able to get the wound closed without skin grafts. Days later and once the infection was treated, we went back to the OR and harvested the paper-thin muscle fascia off the muscle on the side of his upper leg in order to replace the dura since all of it on the affected side had been ripped away during the accident. That would give us a layer to cordon off the brain and spinal fluid from the rest of the repair and let some healing take place. In addition to a resident, the other assist on this case was a licensed surgical assistant and, more important, a PhD anatomist who had spent several hours in the cadaver lab in preparation for this particular case, reviewing the relevant anatomy of the leg muscles, the fascia, and the blood supply. (Later, this individual, Dr. Shane Tubbs, would publish more than a thousand articles in the literature on anatomy and surgery, influence the training of numerous neurosurgeons, and improve the lives of children and adults alike with neurosurgical needs.) The piece of fascia Shane handed up to me harvested from the prepped-out leg was perfectly sized with enough to spare. Nothing could have been more beautiful at the time. We used all of it.

Weeks later, we replaced the portion of the skull that had been pulverized during the trauma or removed during the initial surgery by using layers of Luke's own native skull. It's a method called a split-thickness bone graft and comes from techniques learned from the early twentieth century. When we are under the age of three, the skull is basically thin like a Hershey bar, one layer. This technique, then, of splitting bone, is not an option. As we get older, though, it develops three layers, like an Oreo cookie. (Kids seem to like this analogy when I use it with their parents and they overhear.) So we can harvest a piece of normal skull, then split it with a fine-bladed chisel like separating the layers of an Oreo. Then return the bottom part into its original site and use the harvested top part to cover a bone defect. The plastic polymers that are 3-D-printed, sterilized, and placed in the defects were not an option nearly two decades ago when Luke had his injury. This was the best option at the time.

Once he recovered from the series of reconstructive surgeries, his father relentlessly took him to physical therapy, occupational therapy, and speech therapy, never letting up on him, always at his side. Each time I would see them in clinic in follow-up in the coming months and years, the resultant weakness and speech issues from the initial injury were still present. He had regained limited use of his right arm but could firmly shake hands, was able to walk by adjusting his gait to make up for the weakness in the right leg, and could carry on a simple conversation about rehabilitation and getting back into school. His head shape looked near normal too, only a few patchwork scars under his brown hair. I could feel lumps in the normally smooth contour of the skull, noticeable to no one other than me. He and his father were always so gracious and thankful as I felt around his head for any defects or postoperative healing issues.

For years, I would get photo updates from them, and I can see the last one his father sent me. The boy, in the photo a young man, dressed in a tuxedo for his senior portrait, a smile set on his face. Each time I look at it, I am reminded of when his father and I shared that tiny room in the emergency department. His brain-smeared pants and quiet tears. My pause, then understanding, and my own whispered attempt to tell him, *I will bring him back to you.*

20

Shock Waves

O N THE DAY after her twelfth birthday, my daughter, Fair, handed me a story titled "Bridges" that she had written for a school assignment and asked if I would read it over for her before she turned it in. The following excerpt comes from it directly:

I'm sitting in the back of the class, as usual. I'm trying my hardest not to hear our discussion about the way bridges are built and how they support weight. *I can't think about bridges.*

"Sarah, are you listening?"

No.

I can't say that, though.

"Yes, ma'am."

The teacher gives me a doubtful look.

"What did I say then, Sarah?"

The whole class is staring at me, waiting for my embarrassing answer.

"I . . . I don't know . . . ?"

"I don't tolerate daydreamers in this class, Sarah. I would rather you leave if my discussion is too boring to listen to."

Yes, I know this is a way of teachers to guilt students into feeling bad, but I might as well take my chance and leave early.

I started packing up my things.

"Where are you going? You are not allowed to leave class!"

I ignore her and leave.

And I head to the library.

If you're wondering for a backstory, you're not getting one right now, maybe later.

As I sit at a table, I notice the stack of books next to me. A book sticks out. The title is *Alice in Wonderland*. Of course, it was my sister's favorite book.

Okay, NOW you can get a backstory.

Six months ago, my sister died, due to suicide. She had an Instagram account, where she posted pictures of herself with friends, at the beach, the usual.

Then she started getting comments, saying things like how she was fat, she looked stupid, she wasn't wanted, or she wasn't good enough. And of course, she told people about it, but they told her that she was asking for it and she deserved it for posting pictures of herself in bathing suits.

And of course, she believed them. And didn't tell her family about it. To be honest, I'm going to guess how she was feeling, why she felt she needed to end her life. She was probably confused, for starters. Maybe she felt like she really was stupid, or ugly, or weird. And at the same time, she might also have thought that she really was asking for it, that she shouldn't be sad, she shouldn't be bothered by it. And maybe that made her go down in this pit of feeling and emotions, until she couldn't handle her thoughts anymore and climbed up onto that bridge, jumped and slammed into the water and died. *Did she try to reach back?*

It continues through until finally a resolution of sorts with the bullies, a cleaner version than real life, seen through the eyes of a twelve-year-old, just on the verge of her teenage years. I would imagine that anytime your preteen child writes a story about suicide, it is alarming to parents, as it was initially to us after I shared it with Melissa. We are fortunate that Fair is grounded and emotionally healthy. Still, we, like many others, have a history of mental illness dotted throughout our family, so we are highly keyed in, sometimes overly so. Our concerns were diminished that night at dinner when we brought up her piece. Fair matter-of-factly told us that she had thought about the subject of suicide and social media a good bit lately because she had opened up an Instagram account after her birthday (with our permission) and wanted to be careful and check herself and her friends if things became too intense. She had seen someone talking about cutting on TikTok, and she did *not* want to go there. After a moment to absorb that, we allowed ourselves to be impressed.

"It's like your patient, Dad," said Fair.

"My patient?" I said quietly, and quickly remembered a teenager I had operated on a few years ago who had attempted suicide because of online bullying.

Of course Fair would remember. I had told her an abbreviated and anonymized version of the story at the time. (For the record, it's hard not to bring work home when you are a pediatric neurosurgeon. . . . What once was *Wear your helmet when riding your bike, be careful when you cross the street* has now morphed into *Tell your mother or me if someone you know is talking about harming themselves,* or *If you think of harming yourself because of what people are saying about you online, please* please *talk to us.*)

The story Fair referred to is of a teenage girl named Alyssa, by all accounts attractive and initially popular earlier in elementary school. She received high marks in school, played soccer and softball, and enjoyed hunting with her father, a sheriff's deputy in their small Tennessee town. She was well adjusted, and other than being sassy to her parents from time to time, there was no history of acting out or parental disobedience.

She had occasional issues with her friends but nothing of significance early on. Alyssa was maturing into a beautiful girl and had begun to draw the attention of the boys in her grade. The rivalries with the other girls started out benign enough, but with each school award or recognition one girl group's jealousy moved to malice— soon openly calling her degrading names or mocking photos of her. The forum? Not surprising, the echo chamber of modern social media. Alyssa begged her parents to allow her to change schools. But there were just a few months left in the school year, and her family felt it was best that she face her problems, not run from them, at least until the end of the year. And so she did. Things seemed to quiet down, thankfully, and the rest of the academic year was calm, less dramatic, until the day after school let out for the summer. That day, their family's world changed forever.

I first met Alyssa on the operating room table. It was after midnight when my resident had called me on his way to the operating room as he pushed her gurney up from the ED himself. An ambulance had brought her to our emergency department before her parents, who were still in transit, so I never had the chance to speak to them before surgery. There was no time to get the details of what had happened from the paramedics. As we started to cut her hair away to expose the area for surgery, the long brown locks streaked with blood and bits of bone, someone in the room said that they had heard that a gunman had driven up next to the girl and shot her point-blank through her open car window, assassination style. Something about bullies at her school. I remember a rush of emotion just then, picturing my own kids on the table beneath me.

"Focus, people," I blurted out, louder than I meant to. I started prepping the skin. "None of this matters now. She's on our operating table now, and we have to get her off."

In the OR we cauterized the damaged blood vessels from where the bullet had entered on the right side of her head, the classic right temporal entrance wound of a right-handed person. The trajectory was not from the left as it would be in a driver's-side shooting. The story told earlier was false. I made a quick note of it mentally, *Not the time to talk about it,* and moved on. There was no exit wound, because the bullet had lodged in a thick part of the skull on the left after it had passed through the head. Blood collected underneath the damaged skull on the right side and was under pressure. Without drainage, she would die. Once we removed the bone flap around the bullet hole, drained the blood, and stopped the bleeding, we could see that the bullet had passed through her optic nerves on both sides, immediately blinding her forever. The undersurface of her frontal lobes that overlies the optic nerves was also severely injured, the actual direct penetration injury only a part of the destructive force unleashed by the cavitation from the bullet as it passed through both sides of the brain. Bullets move so fast that they create a pressure wave of air around and just behind them, a shock wave, and it's often that shock wave that causes the most damage as the bullet moves through the tissue.

It was three in the morning when we finished up. The final step was to find her parents and tell them what we had found; I had been taught years ago by a general surgeon during my intern year that speaking with the family after surgery is as much a part of the surgery as the initial incision. No matter if the news was good or bad. Her mother and father had arrived at some point during the night. At the time, I vaguely remembered the circulating nurse taking the call in the OR and telling us.

There were only the two of them in the waiting room at that time in the morning, the next day's patients and parents yet to arrive. They sat huddled together, standing up quickly as I approached them. I hesitated, then pulled up a chair to position myself directly across from them and motioned for them to sit. I then proceeded to tell them that their daughter had survived but that she would forever be blind. The effects of the injury on her brain would take time to be fully known. *The next few days would be crucial.* There was no real way to soften any of it.

I stopped talking and waited. I convinced myself that the most difficult part of the conversation was over. I felt an odd sense of relief begin to come over me.

It was short-lived.

"She shot herself," her mother said, the words coming out between sobs. Both were crying, the father's head buried in his hands.

I remained silent and still across from them.

Her mother continued: "Alyssa's friend"—she stopped to calm herself so that she could get the words out—"said it was something said online."

"I thought that crap was over!" the dad yelled out. "I thought it was over . . ." He trailed off.

They had pieced together what else had happened in the urgent drive to our hospital in the middle of the night.

In a moment's grief, acting out something she had likely walked through in her mind before, she had taken the keys to the family truck out of the kitchen drawer, unlocked the door, then carefully unlocked the glove compartment. There she found her father's service revolver, put it to her head, and fired.

Her father and brother were too far away from the house to hear the shot. Her younger sister is credited with finding her in the truck despite the darkness of night and calling for help. The story is completely finished only when her mother, working at the local 911 dispatch at the time, hears the call for the ambulance urgently needed at her own address.

It was overwhelming to hear, to bear witness to the first telling of the story. I sat for a moment with them. I had no words.

Soon the elevator dinged, and friends and family began to pour out. I stepped away and quietly walked up the nearby stairs, two flights to the ICU. I sat down on a stool next to her bed and waited. *What would she be left with?* I wondered. *Will she be able to comprehend what has happened? What pushed her to this point?*

As I watched her monitor, I let my thoughts drift back to the suicide attempts I had seen in my training while a neurosurgery resident. The images from those days are seared in my mind. I remembered the man in his seventies with a terminal cancer diagnosis who had decided to end his life quickly instead of enduring his worsening pain. After the shotgun blast there was little recognizable left of his face. Even Hollywood at its most macabre could not simulate this level of carnage. His breaths came raspy and began to trail off. I remember the residents on trauma surgery, in my face, yelling about why wasn't I taking this man to the operating room immediately. We were all so young, so pushed to the brink by exhaustion and the dismantling of the world that we thought we knew around us.

As I stood there next to him in that trauma bay, with all the chaos and conflict around me, his blood nearly saturating his pillow, I felt a sense of peace. Peace that I had done what that man wanted. Peace that he had made his choice and we were going to honor that, instead of rushing to try to save him in a futile operation. I came to learn later that he had left a note saying that he wanted to die on his own terms instead of in agony and pumped up on pain medicine. And so he had. I stood next to him and held his hand under the blanket so no one could see me doing it, pretending to examine him, as long as I could. His breath slowed and finally stopped as my pager called me away to some other madness.

Lying there in the hospital bed for weeks, Alyssa initially looked nothing like the photographs of her that her parents taped on the walls around her hospital bed for the medical staff to see who she once was. Her face was swollen, moistened eye dressings in place to reduce the swelling still present in her eyes. She was still unable to close her lids, even reflexively. As the days passed, she slowly began to awaken. Soon she was off the ventilator, the feeding tube had been removed, and she was out of the ICU. Thankfully for her, she could not recall the specific events around her initial presentation to the emergency room, but over time and with recovery she has learned. Her parents were reluctant to tell her, but she kept asking over and over until they finally did, initially only in bits and pieces, each retelling of it like living it over again for them both.

After she was home from the hospital and inpatient rehabilitation, one of the large blood vessels that had been near the shock wave developed an abnormal outpouching, an aneurysm, that was picked up on routine imaging six months after her injury. The blast effect weakened the blood vessel wall just enough so that over time that weakness gave way to the aneurysm. It was not able to be treated from the inside using catheterization and coiling due to its location, so we directly exposed it in an open operation and placed a clip across its neck in the operating room. Even months later, I could see the residual damage from the bullet track directly. I can still see the optic nerves severed on the inside, the internal scar that formed now twisting the surrounding anatomy to something nearly unrecognizable. *What dark place children must go to to push others to this place.* I could not help but see this not as an act of willful self-destruction but as one that Alyssa felt was for self-protection. To get away from the pain. And when it is all around you, as social media can be, it can feel like there is no escape at all. Or at least only one.

Alyssa will forever live with the profound effects of that day. Both she and her parents wanted her story told so that people might understand that social bullying is real. Her mom asked me to make sure that people understand that Alyssa has worked hard since that day to be a good young woman living out her faith. For all that she has endured, Alyssa loves the idea of being able to help others, and that is how she understands her purpose now. She does not remember much of her life before her injury. But she makes a point to say that we sometimes can inflict pain on one another without much thought. It can be awful. And then she says she knows that we can do better.

21

Closure

OTHER THAN AS the target of a lawsuit, a doctor has two other main reasons to interact with the medical malpractice world. The first and most straightforward is as a treating physician to help explain to a judge or jury a particular aspect of a patient's medical condition or clinical course. This we are obligated to do, and appropriately so. Testimony here may be critical in order to understand what the issues were surrounding a particular clinical decision, why such-and-such surgery was done, or how the person will be forever affected. Many times for us as pediatric neurosurgeons this testimony is in the context of non-accidental trauma, where an injury to a child is committed by an adult and our role is to say what a traumatic subdural hematoma is, why it's an emergency, and what the long-term impact might be for the child's development. The effects of being harmed purposely by someone who is meant to care for you can be quite profound—lifelong, permanent. Also profound is the degree to which many other lives are affected when this happens: parent, sibling, extended family, and abuser.

The other reason is to act as an expert witness (a.k.a. a hired gun) who is contacted by either of the legal teams in a civil case, or the prosecution or defense in a criminal case, to review the facts and render an opinion, usually around whether the "standard of care" was met. This can be formally delivered in a video deposition, during which both sides ask questions and have the right to object, and is certified by the presence of a court reporter. Stepping into the role of expert witness can also find a doctor on the stand in the courtroom during the legal case itself. *Clearly the surgeon's decision to perform such-and-such surgery did not meet the standard of care.* There is a whole career to be made here.

I have never chosen to do this. Partially because I have had other, more pressing things to take care of in addition to patient care, mostly administrative or educational or research based.

But that is all just a convenient excuse, because I have never had the desire to press my surgical opinion upon someone else or cast judgment on what someone has done or not done. Experience has taught me that often there are several alternatives to how a situation—especially a dire emergency—can be approached. Indeed, as a surgeon and a pilot's son I often think about the military concept called the "fog of war" and how often a decision must be made in the moment without the benefit of the calm and information available in hindsight. All of it makes me hesitant to pass judgment. *Judge not, lest yourselves be judged* is also on my mind. I'm not eager to have any of my less than ideal outcomes aired in a public forum. My attorney friends say "whatever" and tell me that I am the definition of how the medical system fails to police itself. In some ways they are correct.

One thing I seem to have no problem with whatsoever is self-criticism. I can keep myself quite busy with examining my own actions, sometimes reaching a near-constant state of self-reflection. This self-criticism, I suspect, has little to do with my being a doctor; if I were an English professor or a shoe salesman, I would be similarly self-critical. I do concede that the consequences of misgrading a paper or giving poor advice on an instep might be orders of magnitude different from surgical errors. But neurosurgery is *hard,* and there is not always the exact right answer. As my residents have heard me say many times, there is very little in our field that you turn to page 342 in the book of pediatric neurosurgery to find the answer for.

I held to this practice of not passing judgment in my rare engage-ments with the legal system for many years until an unforgettable encounter with a patient several years ago. But even then, I never had the full story. I was perfectly content to leave it in the past.

IN ADDITION TO operating on brain and spinal cord issues, a subset of neurosurgeons operate on the peripheral nerves. These nerves link the central nervous system to all the muscles in order to ini-tiate and control movement or carry sensation like touch or posi-tion or pain from the skin or deeper parts of the body. That pain can be slight and irritative, or it can be deep and electric shock–like and unrelenting. Nerves can be compressed over time, carpal tun-nel syndrome being the most common form of this. Compression causes weakness, numbness, or pain anywhere in the body, depend-ing on the nerve involved. Severe nerve trauma from a car accident, a gunshot wound, or a knife injury can also occur to just about any peripheral nerve as well. Whereas adults tend to be the ones who develop the compression issues over time, children are more likely to suffer traumatic injury than compression. If the injured nerve is stretched but not severely, then in the vast majority of cases the function returns over months. On occasion, the nerve can be sev-ered, and the ramifications of that can be profound in a life-altering, never-ending, don't-touch-me kind of way.

More than a decade ago, I stood outside one of the rooms in my clinic and read the chart. "Leg weakness and pain." I read further. He was eleven years old, and the pain was in both legs. As I looked through the records from the outside referring primary care doctor, I saw that the symptoms had been there for months. *Why hadn't any-one ordered a spine MRI yet?* I wondered, since both legs were involved and that usually meant a more central process. I began to imagine that this family, who had traveled from five hours away, would be annoyed at having to get an MRI, so I thought through my words carefully before I headed in. Soon, all of that wouldn't matter.

When I opened the door, I found the lights dim and the boy curled up in a ball on the examining table. There was no movement, no greeting. He lay still and his parents sat in the chairs watching him. There was an overwhelming sense of pain in the room. Pain with movement, pain with examination, pain with living. The type of pain that suffuses everyone and everything around the patient. Both parents were there, and a grandmother. Everyone quiet, moving as little as possible. As I entered, I noticed that the boy was under a blanket, his hips turned to the wall, and that his eyes were closed. For the next thirty minutes, I examined him as best I could, trying to minimize the agony that he felt with even the slightest movement of his legs. We weren't prepared for a child to be experiencing this type of pain in an outpatient consult clinic. We had graham crackers and Buzz Lightyear stickers, little help here. I considered sending him to the emergency department for help. Then his mother slipped him a pill from an unmarked bottle in her purse and soon he had calmed down. His breathing slowed, his eyes closed, and then mercifully, he slept.

From his parents I heard how he had been an athlete, a soccer player, and had been noted to have a slight degree of leg "tightness" on both sides; the parents used air quotes when they said this. *Best to see someone about some therapy,* they were told. *Focused stretching might help.* Initially, he was referred to a local physical therapy group who suggested a series of exercises and leg stretches for him to do. It was also recommended that he see an orthopedic surgeon as part of the protocol for children with spasticity—the medical term for muscle tightness that can be due to any number of reasons. Most commonly, the actual cause is unknown and thought to be due to an injury in utero or during birth. When the family met with the surgeon, in addition to the therapy he was receiving, it was recommended that he undergo surgery to loosen the tendons of his hamstrings behind the knees—by cutting them under general anesthesia in the operating room. They were surprised, but after a discussion and assurances that the procedure was in his best interest and the most effective way to get him back to the soccer field, the family had agreed, expecting an outpatient procedure that would have him recovered and back to sports in six weeks. It was explained how he would awaken after surgery with his legs casted in a straighter position. But he would be running in no time.

Instead, several months had passed since his operation, and here he was.

He called out again from his sleep. The stirring causing him to wake up from the pain. The parents' attention immediately went to the boy.

"Hey, Seymore, it's okay, buddy," his father said, gently smoothing his hair, "it's okay." We waited for a bit, and once he was asleep again, they continued.

After that surgery, Seymore woke up with leg casts on both sides from his knees down. The first thing the parents noted was the significant pain he was in, wildly reaching out in the recovery room, thrashing about, yelling. Despite this, he was discharged and the family reassured that his reaction was normal. At home, he was exactly the same when the pain medicine would wear off. When the time came days later for physical therapy, he was completely incapable of participating. After a month, still casted, he was barely able to bring one foot in front of the other using a walker. When the casts were finally cut away, he was found to have no movement in his ankles or toes. He was also numb from the knees down. Worse, he was developing unrelenting pain. And it would only get worse.

There was no spine MRI needed here. This had nothing to do with the spinal cord or a more central process that I had hypothesized outside the door. With his combination of symptoms, it gradually began to dawn on me what had happened. The boy must have had major nerve damage—*on both sides.* I assumed damaged during the operation. *What in the world happened?*

There is a huge nerve, in adults nearly as thick as the thumb, that runs down the back of the upper leg, hidden deep in the muscles. This nerve, the sciatic nerve, then passes behind the knee, splitting into two parts that continue into the lower leg. One part of the nerve passes into the muscles of the calf and enables us to push our feet down against the ground, allowing us to propel ourselves through space. The other part of the nerve curves around the outside of the leg and runs to the muscles on the front of the lower leg. These muscles allow us to pull our foot and toes up to complete the motion of walking.

As I examined the boy as best I could, it was clear to me that he could not move either foot, or feel sensation in his lower legs below the knees, and had significant shock-like pain that worsened with movement. Pain like that is called neuropathic pain and is a sign that the nerves are somehow involved. *Perhaps,* I rationalized to myself, *there could be scar formation around the nerves causing the pain,* completely disregarding the fact that he woke up like this after surgery. Scar doesn't form that early. Regardless, the only way to help was to explore the affected areas. With another surgery. On both sides.

In the meantime, we brought Seymore's pain down as best we could with the help of our rehabilitation doctor and our pain team. I was very straightforward with Seymore's parents when talking about the proposed surgery. I had not seen a nerve injury of this magnitude before, and the fact that it was on both sides was mind-boggling. I had operated on the sciatic nerve several times, but this would be different. We would start higher up the back of the leg than the scarred area because I assumed the normal anatomy would be thrown off there. Prior surgery tends to do that, distort the normal anatomy, sometimes a great deal and sometimes just enough to throw off typical relationships. In order to make our way through this, we would need to start well above and well below the area of injury, in normal tissue, to find the nerve and make our way down. I told all of this to the family. What I did not tell them was that I had begun to suspect that the nerves had been cut clean through alongside the muscle tendons, perhaps even instead of the tendons. My mind could see that relationship. But I was not certain what had happened. I was yet to see it with my own eyes.

Many years ago, as a chief resident, I remember coming into my chairman's office late at night to "run the list" with him, where the two of us would review the status of his patients and update any plans before we both headed home. Any changes I could relate to the on-call resident or stay and accomplish myself if necessary. I remember thinking that I was assisting him with a challenging surgery the next day, but not being surprised to see him there so late. I had given up trying to understand his schedule long ago.

I entered the room outside his office quietly. The door to his inner office was cracked open, and he did not look up. I peered through, stealing a moment to watch him in the same way I had observed him in the operating room all those times. He was carefully flipping the pages of an anatomy textbook and reviewing the area we were going to be operating on the next day. I remember being amazed that this person who asked me anatomy question after question in each case I performed with him was reviewing that same anatomy the night before. I thought that knowledge was just always in there—*in your brain*—once you reach a certain point. But that was not right. After two decades, I certainly know that now. But I learned that night that a surgeon always needed to review beforehand, particularly for the rare or less encountered cases. Since that very moment watching my chairman through the crack in the opened door, I spend the last few minutes at my desk on the nights before operations reviewing the anatomy. It has become a ritual. I've walked back up nine flights of stairs to my office to do it when I had forgotten and the elevator was moving too slow. That night before Seymore's surgery, I spent well more time than normal.

In the OR, we initially explored the right leg behind the knee. After parting the muscle bellies of the hamstrings and carefully protecting the large artery and vein signaling the nearby presence of our intended nerve, we came to the sciatic nerve as it exited from the muscle in the upper leg and followed it along its course. From there, we made our way farther down the leg through the prior scar. The tissue was indeed thickened, difficult to dissect through. There was a little more bleeding than if the area had been untouched. As we continued moving through the area, slower than normal, we found that instead of the nerve continuing on into the lower leg, it ended in a bulbous ball of scar tissue. Next to the nerve, perhaps one centimeter away, was the intact hamstring tendon, the intended target of the initial surgery. The nerve had been cut during the prior surgery instead of the tendon.

We then went below the knee, made an incision, and found the two distal nerves where they traveled into both the front and the back of the leg. Then we followed them both up until the nerves just ended blindly. Again, one centimeter away was the intact hamstring tendon.

My resident and I looked at each other, both quiet, both aghast at what we were seeing. The sciatic nerve, just above its split, had been severed completely. In its place, an ugly bulbous neuroma on the proximal end, where the tiny microscopic individual nerve processes had tried to grow back, probing randomly across the gap for the other side. Over time those nerve processes matted up into a ball of scar tissue that is nonfunctional and often extremely painful when jostled. The nerves above and below the injury had to be cut back to more normal-appearing tissue, ultimately resulting in an even wider gap between the proximal and the distal nerves. In an effort to repair the damage we'd found by providing a series of conduits for the nerves, we harvested the sural nerve from the side of the leg. The sural nerve is a long thin nerve around the diameter of the low E guitar string, and it gives sensation only to a small area on the lateral foot. There is no movement associated with it at all. At some point in my career, possibly here, I started calling it God's gift to the peripheral nerve surgeon because of its generous length and because cutting it results in no motor deficits. Perfect to be used for grafting. Seymore had no sensation in the entire foot at this point anyway, so he would not be able to tell in the long run.

We measured the gap and cut the long sural nerve into six shorter segments so that we could sew multiple cable grafts across the gap. We used suture the size of human hair and the operating microscope in order to adequately visualize what we were doing. The entire procedure took several hours to accomplish, including closing the two long incisions on the back of his leg that exposed both the sciatic injury and the separate sural nerve harvesting, but all went fine. When the morning first began, I had considered repairing the damage to both legs. When I saw the magnitude of the situation, I realized that was hubris. Eight hours after we had begun the initial exploration, we were done.

A few days later, we brought Seymore back to the OR for the left side, finding a similar severed nerve and neuroma at the same place in the leg, as well as the intact hamstring. I reconstructed the nerve in the same way, except the gap on this side was slightly longer, and the sural nerve was not quite long enough to give the number of segments we needed. I found a nearby vein and used that, having read in preparation for the operation that it was possible to use it in a pinch. Two days later, Seymore was home in his own bed. It would be months before we would know whether the grafts took. Repairing nerves is not like rewiring a lamp. The axons die back to the spinal cord, leaving the tiny channels of myelin intact. Slowly, sprouting off the spinal cord, the axons grow back, one millimeter a day. When the group of axons finally make their way down to the gap, they look for guidance, be it the leftover microscopic tunnels or even that nearby vein sewn in. It can be six to nine months before you know if a single nerve graft in the leg is working because there is such a long way to travel, let alone twelve of them. So we all settled in for a long wait. Despite the significance of the damage, I was hopeful.

At the two-week post-op check, I took a moment to steel myself outside the clinic door before I walked in. I remembered how much pain there was the last time I had seen him in this room. This time, Seymore was sitting up in a chair. The lights were on and the family was laughing at a joke he had told right before I walked in. He was off pain medicine completely. It was a remarkable transformation. Even with no change in function at this point, the absence of pain made a tremendous difference. Later, at six months, he flexed an ankle. At seven months, both ankles flexed and extended, and he wiggled his big toe. The last time I saw him, eighteen months after the surgery, he was weak but walking, and with a degree of sensation back in his feet. He showed me that he could stand up on his tiptoes. It was amazing to see, and well more than I had hoped for. He had clearly regained a significant amount of movement and strength, and on both sides. He proudly told me that he had played a game of soccer with his friends. His parents sat behind him, smiling broadly.

"Tell my Seymore to wear those ankle braces you gave him, Dr. Wellons," said his mother. "He just kicks them off and keeps on going."

"It just makes my scars itch, Momma," he said as he reached around to rub the scars running down the backs of both legs. "Beside, I don't need them."

During that last visit, as we were winding down, his mother asked me the question that I had been expecting in some form for some time.

"You think we should sue that other doctor, don't you, Dr. Wellons? This shouldn't have happened. It was so different from what we were told."

To the layman, this seems obvious. To me at the time, I felt as if I were standing over an abyss, about to recommend legal action where I felt for many years that I was in no place to judge the actions of others. *The nerve was so close to the hamstring, after all.*

Then I thought about that very first visit. How his father had smoothed his son's hair after he had cried out.

Hey, Seymore, it's okay, buddy.

This family of limited resources had stopped their whole world to find help for their son. He was indeed getting better, but despite that he would never fully be the same. I gently inquired if they had spoken to a lawyer. They had not, she said. They wanted my opinion. They wanted to know what I would do if it were my own child. A question that would focus me for my entire career. One that immediately snaps me to attention, that demands that I speak the truth.

Hey, Seymore, it's okay, buddy.

"Yes," I said. "Yes, if it were my son, I would speak with a lawyer. There are ways to help secure help for him and for you all moving forward."

We continued to talk. I offered to do whatever I could to help them. That meant providing testimony on what I had seen in the operations and what my conclusions were. To some extent I felt I would rely on the old legal adage *res ipsa loquitur,* the thing speaks for itself.

Before I left the exam room, I looked at Seymore and told him he would keep getting better and that we were all very proud of him.

Then, before I knew it, the words spilled out of my mouth.

"No matter what happens, Seymore, you are not to think of yourself as less capable than anyone else. This is just part of your life, something put in your path to overcome.

"Promise me that," I said to him. I looked at his parents, who looked at their son. His father had tears in his eyes.

THE VIDEO DEPOSITION took place one morning months later in a hospital conference room, the sun pouring through the blinds. There were several photographs that I had taken during surgery that were used as evidence, blown up and turned into large posters on easels. As both sides asked me questions, I kept focusing on that boy curled up in a ball on my examining table when all of this began. Over the course of my life in medicine, many of the things that have stuck with me are my own mistakes. I have a deep fear of being called out on them. *You did not prepare enough. You did not try hard enough. You had no business doing that procedure. How could you pass judgment?* But those voices were quiet. This felt very different.

As the lawyers continued, I heard for the very first time how the family was chastised for their questions after the first surgery, when, instead of healing, their son was in debilitating pain. Short notes from the prior surgeon's office chart painted the family out to be overreacting and malingering, in plain view on the official copy of the medical record in front of me. The plaintiff's attorney asked me to read several of the notes aloud for the court record, implying that they were whiners or seeking pain medicine. I was dumbfounded.

In the first year of my practice, I approached a wise adult vascular neurosurgeon partner whom I admired named Wink Fisher to obtain advice as I was starting out as an attending. Wink was experienced in the world of operating on the extremely ill, with a lifetime of pulling some back from over the edge and having to let some of them go. He told me that when I had a complication or unexpected negative outcome after surgery, *And you will, Jay, because if you do this long enough, we all do,* instead of running away from the patient or family, you actually needed to lean in closer to them. So that they feel your presence and know that you are in it with them, as far as they will have you. Those words of advice have stayed with me to this day.

But to hear that a surgeon had mocked a suffering patient, when he himself had caused that suffering? And to dismiss this family whom I had spent so much time with, whom I had walked this journey with? I felt anger. Anger that burned away any last remaining restraint I might have felt. Once the deposition was over, I had a difficult time hiding my disdain for the defense attorney team.

I heard weeks later that the case had been settled. I chose to not learn any more of the details than that. I just held on to the narrative that Seymore continued to improve and that a measure of justice had been achieved. A happy ending. On to the next patient. I had done my part.

And there this story stayed for a decade. For the intervening years, I pictured that young man growing older, holding a job, his parents settled in their retirement. I hoped that he had put those days of curled-up darkness and pain long behind him, and that every once in a while, when he felt the ridges of the scars on his legs, he would have to focus to remember why they were there at all. In all the later cases of nerve injury that I took care of afterward, I would think back to this one story, recounting at least part of it to my residents or students in the operating room or in lectures. *All worked out fine for him,* I would think to myself. *It must have.*

Recently, one of my residents asked me if I ever knew what became of Seymore as he grew into adulthood. The question awakened the memory and kept coming back to me over and over. In the past, I would convince myself that I would rather have the memory of the potential for a normal life, rather than find out the opposite. Then, just as in my response to the family's question about legal intervention in the exam room at that eighteen-month follow-up visit, I changed my mind. I decided to reach out to them and find out what Seymore's life had become all these years later.

After some research, I found his parents' telephone number.

More than a decade had gone by, and I had no idea what to expect. I picked up the telephone, partially dialing the number at least ten times before I was actually able to force myself to complete the call.

Seymore's mother picked up. I immediately recognized her voice. The feeling of taking care of him flooded back to me: the pre-op visits, the discussions after surgery, the follow-ups. Both the hard conversations beforehand and the joyous ones when he was clearly getting better. There was a shared history that she and I had lived together. I could hear my voice betraying my nervousness.

There was a pause after I reintroduced myself.

"Oh my heavens, it's Dr. Wellons!" she said. "Everybody!" she called out. "It's Dr. Wellons!" I heard commotion in the background. "Oh, you would be so proud. Seymore is twenty-one years old. He finished high school without any assistance and works as a mechanic fixing helicopters on a nearby army base. He's there right now in fact. He works hard and Seymore makes a good living for himself," she said proudly. She went on to tell me that he was happy, walking or driving "anywhere he wants.

"And he still isn't wearing those braces you gave him," she said. We laughed together. The sheer joy of it all was wonderful.

After a while, the conversation drifted to the results of the legal case. She went on to tell me that the lawyers that had taken their case had to come from a town nearly a hundred miles away. All the legal firms they had talked to near where they lived had conflicts or were on retainer for the defense. I had had no idea. Rather than go to court, where the surgeon would have certainly been convicted of malpractice, the defense ultimately settled, due to my testimony, she said. The surgeon never admitted in public his responsibility for the severed nerves, but the family thought the settlement was fair.

Then she continued. It turned out that the surgeon involved was found to be writing illegal opioid prescriptions and had temporarily lost his medical license. Later it was reported in the news that he had voluntarily surrendered his license for good for alleged inappropriate conduct with patients. With this sudden full knowledge, I found it particularly ironic that I had been at all reluctant to suggest they get a lawyer all those years ago.

"Things like this have a way of working out," Seymore's mom said. "We were all just feeling our way through the dark. I'm so glad we did what we did. We knew what happened to him shouldn't have.

"Seymore doesn't need any help with his life," she added. "He's never lived like he was different from anybody else." She paused. Her voice began to crack. "He did just what you said that very last day we saw you."

I could hear her crying now as she said, "You'd be so proud of him. Somehow he's managed to come out stronger than we'd ever even imagined."

22

The Other Side

SEVERAL YEARS AGO, after a particularly busy week in the operating room, I waited impatiently at my desk at work after rounds
on a Saturday morning for a contrasted brain MRI to be performed
on an eighteen-year-old boy whom I had operated on the previous
afternoon for the second time in two days. He had presented with a
series of odd-shaped cavernomas in the back of his brain—a chain
of them to be exact—that were off to the left and taking up much
of the cerebellum on that side, abutting the brainstem, and jutting
out into an area just outside them both called the cerebellopon-
tine angle, rich with critical blood vessels and nerves. The morning
prior, as the image scrolled across my screen in real time just like
now, I could clearly see what was left. The deepest part. His lesion,
a cerebral cavernoma, like Allie's except on the outside and inside
of the cerebellum and lateral brainstem, instead of entirely inside
the pons, like hers.

Sometimes they never change in size or shape, and never require
surgery. But some have them and they grow, or compress an important part of the brain, or cause seizures, or even rupture in a life-
threatening way. This boy's cavernoma had been operated on years
ago by another surgeon for an acute rupture. It was a lifesaving
emergency, and back then part of it was left because it was decided
it was too difficult to resect. Too much risk. And there it stayed for

several years without changing until recently, when it enlarged, significantly, the trigger unknown.

Even now, after twenty years, it is not uncommon for me to be "a little" impatient each time I wait on a postoperative MRI to be done. What waits to be seen on that scan has tremendous ramifications for the patient and their parents. For both them and the surgeon it is a signal of success or failure—*did you get it all?*—and it is intimately intertwined with the other determinant: How the child wakes up after surgery. How they interact with the world around them. *Did we go too far?* Did we injure them in the process? Did we walk the exact fine line necessary to rid them of whatever menace brought them here yet also manage to keep all the higher brain functions intact so that the family can take home someone similar to the person they brought to me?

Years ago, in my first month of practice, when the true weight of being a fully trained pediatric neurosurgeon finally dawned on me, I sat with my senior partner Jerry Oakes with my head in my hands after rendering a young girl aphasic—unable to speak—from an operation to remove a tumor abutting the speech area. That postoperative scan was clean of tumor, but it took her a day—a very long never-encountered-by-me-before day—to recover enough of her speech for us to know she would ultimately be all right. As I sat there in his office, nervously rubbing my hands, I'm not sure what I expected him to say. Some balm perhaps. Some story of his first days as a surgeon.

Jerry sat there for a minute, looked up at me from his desk, and said, "Welcome to the big leagues."

So there I was once again reflecting about being in the big leagues, now having swung twice at this previously unresectable lesion, waiting again to see what the scan would look like. As with many things I have experienced in my two decades of being a pediatric neurosurgeon, the story behind the re-resection goes a bit deeper than simply residual lesion and a take-back operation.

Hayden was the young man's name. When I had spoken to him and his parents about the risks of having to go right back again to the OR, now for a third time including that initial resection so long ago, his mother began to gently cry. I suppose it would be easy to judge me because I had to take him back. *I did not get it all out. He will have to undergo the risk of surgery again. I am desperately sorry.* (Believe me, there is a voice inside me saying that exact same thing for some reason or another, 24/7.) Indeed, there are now hospital metrics for returns to the OR, called RTOR, that are tracked by a clipboard-wielding administrator, nurse, or doctor whose sole purpose is to measure quality metrics. Think ERA, earned run average, but for a surgeon, not a pitcher—the lower, the better. We are expected to have as few take backs as possible. Insurance companies reduce the amount paid for the second surgery, so hospital finance leaders dislike it when they have to be done. Not surprisingly, parents like it even less. And to be clear, I'm not a fan, either.

My relationship with this particular family goes back quite some time. I'd been seeing Hayden and his parents every year in clinic for the eight years since I had arrived in Nashville. Each year he was a little taller, a little more mature, always with a "yes, sir" and a strong handshake. At the last visit, Hayden had proudly told me about a job he had working construction in the summers, using his hands, learning to build houses from the foundation up. He was proud to swing a hammer and had been moved up to a nail gun the previous summer. So his balance, strength, and reaction time were all sources of pride to him, something never taken for granted because he remembered enough of his early days recovering after that long-ago surgery to know not to.

His brain MRI had been stable since I had first met him in clinic. But for all the years I had seen him in follow-up, down low on the scan and off to the left, he had a stable, oddly shaped blood vessel malformation, the size of a small marble, embedded in his brainstem near the takeoff of the seventh and eighth nerves (which control movement on the left side of your face, hearing, and balance). As mentioned, his cavernoma had not changed since the last surgeon's post-op scan years before. His parents had no interest in going back for a full resection in the years afterward. Hayden had "taken a hit"—meaning suffered a neurologic injury—with that initial hemorrhage and subsequent life-saving procedure, and it had taken time to recover. Now he was neurologically intact and liked the idea of staying that way. Surgery was long ago. He and his parents were well past it. They had fallen into the familiar rhythm of yearly scans with no change. They had fallen into thinking that they were past it, on to the other side.

I had, too.

A few weeks before, I had seen his name on my clinic list for the day and had been looking forward to seeing him and his parents and to hearing about his next steps in life. Hayden was eighteen. All had been stable for so long. With luck, one day, all these visits and all these scans would be a distant memory.

I read over my last office note from more than a year ago. Then I pulled up his MRI from earlier that morning while swilling my coffee. I learned many years ago to not let too much time go by between getting the actual MRI and telling the patient's parents what it shows. Oftentimes now it's the first thing I say when I walk into the room.

What I saw in that clinic visit on that computer screen stopped me mid-drink. The change was not subtle. I placed my cup on the edge of the desk and sat down in the nearest chair.

The cavernoma had grown. And not just a little, but a lot. Instead of a small marble, the lesion was now five times its previous size and was displacing the surrounding brain and nerves. Somehow it had just let loose since the last scan a year before.

As if that itself weren't enough, several more lesions had popped up in Hayden's cerebellum, like little stepping-stones leading from the surface down deeper and deeper to the largest one embedded in the lateral brainstem. The deepest one had grown enough to break through the surface of the brainstem, only its thin wall itself keeping the blood inside. As with Allie, surgery was the only answer.

As I sat outside the clinic door and scrolled the mouse wheel watching the images flash across the screen in sequence, all I could think about was what I was about to say when I walked into the room.

When you see a new patient's scan for the first time, usually before a consult in the ED or clinic, the images are sterile, devoid of the human being depicted, devoid of any humanity at all. It is for that brief moment simply a problem to be solved. A problem that is yet to be suffused with the suffering and understandable anxiety that a neurosurgical diagnosis can bring. It can be a pause allowing clarity that helps to map out a plan in your own brain on what must be done to bring the situation to resolution. It is critically important to have a plan for parents and patients—*There is peace with a plan,* as my now chairman Reid Thompson espouses—because it begins the turn from the unknown to the known.

Once you meet the patient and family, the equation changes. The issue represented on the screen is no longer academic, no longer distant. The images become secondary to the person. Instead of being identified in your own thoughts as the CT scan showing the fractured lower spine that needs to go to the OR later today, the situation becomes the six-year-old boy in the PICU who loves to climb trees with his sister. Instead of the MRI showing a Chiari I malformation, soon it will change into the fifteen-year-old girl in clinic who can no longer pitch a softball due to debilitating headaches and wants to play college ball. The open depressed skull fracture on the computer screen becomes the two-year-old girl in the trauma bay of the emergency department who had been on her way to daycare with her father when someone turned quickly in front of them. Despite all this, the pain, the grief, the anxiety (and the projection I cannot help but have), it is key to the role of neurosurgeon to be the person who brings a solution if there is one to be had. Whether an emergency or a long-term plan, parents need to hear the next steps, to regain even the slightest amount of balance in their world that has been turned upside down.

Hayden and his parents knew something was wrong, even before I opened the clinic door. They all had suspected something in the weeks beforehand; he had started to lose coordination in his left hand. They all knew, even if they didn't speak of it with one another. He had gotten up from the dinner table the week before enraged, unable to cut his steak because of the tremor in his hand. His chair bounced off the floor as he charged up to his room while the rest of the family ate in silence.

If it were my child, I would want to know immediately. I have a terrible poker face. I'm unable to go through pleasantries when there is something to tell that will be hard to hear. And so without a moment's pause, before we had exchanged greetings, not even taking the time to sit down, I said, "Hello, everybody, it's gotten bigger."

Then, in that moment, when everyone looked down to gather their thoughts and steel themselves for their new reality, I stepped in closer to examine Hayden. The new dyscoordination was on full display. There was no question Hayden was worse. I asked him to reach out with his right hand for a pen in my hand. Smooth. No problem. But with his left hand, he was all over the place. Because of the tremor, he was unable to grab the pen normally with that hand. Finally he reached out with his normal right hand and took the pen and handed it to his left hand. I pulled up the images on the computer to show them. For this part, we send some kids out of the room. The surgery discussion can be scary. Risks have to be reviewed. But not with Hayden. I knew to not even ask. He wanted to be there, to understand. I just launched right into it. *There is peace with a plan.*

When I was done talking them all through it, both Mom and

Dad were stone-faced. They remained seated and looked up at their son.

Hayden, who had been leaning against the examination table and staring at his left hand as I explained the plan, calmly looked at me and said, "Doc, I want you to get it out."

"I will, Hayden—" I started to answer, but he cut me off.

"But if you get to a point where this is too deep in there, I want you to stop."

The comment hung there for a moment.

I remained silent, not sure how to proceed. Then he continued.

"There's no shame in stopping and coming back, Doc," he said. "You've been looking after me for a long time now."

He paused to look at me, then said, "I trust you." Then, looking at his parents, he said, "My parents do too."

Dumbfounded and amazed at their son, they looked over to me and nodded their heads.

He continued, "If you need to stop, do that MRI, and come back with another operation, then so be it. Whatever you need to do to fix this. Don't get me wrong, I want it out, but I want the other side of this to be a place where I can be outside framing a house, hammering, whatever, just using my hands." He paused, then said, "I need to be able to use my hands."

He looked away to the window.

I was stunned by his maturity. Such calmness and matter-of-factness in the face of what he had heard only minutes before but had suspected for much longer. Most of my patients were much younger. This was not the same as handing out stickers in clinic or sitting at the bedside telling a young child the overly simplified *we are going to take out what is hurting you and help you get better*. This young man was giving me permission to back out if things weren't clear. To let the dust settle, get a post-op image, and come back if we needed to. RTOR clipboards and metrics be damned.

In the operating room a few days later, the scarred area from the surgery years earlier made it challenging to follow our plan. I could not get a consistent read on the anatomy. Over the years, scar had formed in Hayden's cerebellum, the relationships of crucial structures altered. Under the operating microscope and using the intraoperative ultrasound, we finally found the first cavernoma and made our way in, deeper, resecting each lesion one by one, as best we could until we were staring at the main cavernoma next to the takeoff from the brainstem of the seventh and eighth nerves. Both were plastered to the surface of the cavernoma. Both nerves are fragile, prone to injury if the slightest movement becomes too vigorous. In this tiny world, too vigorous is judged by millimeters. I tried to dissect them away from the side of the brainstem. A claxon from the corner of the room. It was the nerve monitor. We monitor both of the delicate nerves during these cases, and the slightest injury can cause permanent damage to the ability to close the eyelid or open the mouth or hear. I backed out. I then found the side of the cavernoma and opened it up. Again, the alarms sounded, for longer than I'd like, indicating possible lasting damage. *Damn it, we are losing facial nerve function.*

The seventh cranial nerve comes out of the lateral brainstem and carries the signal from the brain to move the face at will. The nerve is also extremely sensitive to manipulation, particularly when it is stretched thin across the surface of a brain tumor, most commonly, or other lesion that shouldn't be there. Too vigorous a dissection and the entire left side of his face would be paralyzed.

I decided that we would wait a bit and try again. If the alarm recedes, then the risk for permanent damage decreases, and we can start back in. We irrigated, the tiny arc of sterile fluid bathing and calming the sensitive and irritated nerve. The monitoring alarm slowed and then silenced, telling us that the facial nerve function had recovered. We start back dissecting. Again, the alarm. Again, I irrigated. The cycle repeated twice more.

"Dr. Wellons?" tentatively said the resident assisting me. This is a particularly hard case, so most of her learning today comes from watching. She says this next part so that only I can hear her. "I feel like this is where you should be telling me that we should stop."

And of course, she was right.

So we stopped. We stopped, knowing that we would likely need to come back. I thought about Hayden's words to me from a few days before.

I trust you. My parents trust you.

After the next day's MRI confirmed what we knew, that there was indeed residual cavernoma left, I spoke to the family and said we would go back to the OR later that same day. We had an open room and an anesthetic team available. Since the nerve was so sensitive, this time we would try an approach from a slightly different angle. I thought that would allow us the best chance of doing something different from the last time so that we could do what we came to do.

The difference a change can make in positioning a patient's head at a certain angle, or entering in along a different trajectory, is remarkable, akin to taking a completely different road to your same destination. As the tiny structures rotate, even a few degrees, the relationship of one to the other changes. Under the operating microscope, that change can make the difference between getting a tumor or cavernoma out and not, between too much traction on a cranial nerve and not, between not seeing the back side of a blood vessel and mistakenly tearing it open. Soon, Hayden was anesthetized again, and we were back in the same place from that ever-so-slightly different angle, trying to flank it from the outside in. There, just around an area of scarred brain, lay the cavernoma, a purple bulging of dilated and abnormal thin-walled veins, pushing itself into the space outside the brain. We could trace the scarred-down seventh and eighth nerves well enough, the entire course of them wrapped around the cavernoma and passing through the internal auditory meatus, the term for the internal hole in the ear that communicates to the brain cavity. (The external auditory meatus is its better-known partner, known as the outer ear canal.)

Under the microscope, the cavernoma looked like two blackberries side by side. It was not obvious if we had even had any effect on this final lesion in the chain from the surgery the day before. One part in the brainstem, the other between the seventh and the eighth nerves. It was much clearer approaching from this direction. We carefully opened the lateral membrane of the cavernoma nestled in between the nerves, drained the blood, and carefully cut the walls away from the nerves using the microscissors—the whole time being careful not to trigger the monitors. This released the traction on the nerves that had been upsetting the monitors before. The monitors went off briefly, but just as quickly trailed off.

I spent half an hour scouring the resection cavity, trying to see if there was any residual cavernoma left. At the end, I saw nothing. The brain pulsated the slightest amount with each heartbeat. Just as it should. The spinal fluid was clear, no sign of hemorrhage from an unseen bleeding vessel at all. It was time to close up. I persuaded myself to look again. Finally, there was no place else to look. It was clean; there was no residual cavernoma, at least that I could see. We closed up. The dura was closed with a tight running suture line, bone flap replaced, and skin sutured up. The resident placed a dressing on the incision and a head wrap around the operative area.

Then we waited on Hayden to wake up.

To our surprise, he came out of his third round of anesthesia in forty-eight hours (OR, MRI, then OR again) better than he had gone in. Not only was his facial movement preserved, but his left-hand coordination had actually improved. Not a little but a lot. He gave me a thumbs-up with both arms from the gurney as he rolled up to the ICU. I was hopeful but guarded with the family about the scan scheduled for the next morning.

* * *

WHICH BRINGS ME back to my desk on a Saturday morning, just after rounds, waiting. Waiting on the scan. Sleep came on and off the night prior. Some from on-call consults. Some from "pre-living" this moment. It has been the same way for years for me. All else fading to the background, the wait becoming nearly intolerable as the time comes closer. *Let the scan be clean. Please.*

I refreshed the screen again. Pause.

Still nothing.

I called down to the MRI control room. *He's on the table, Dr. Wellons. Be patient,* they tell me, laughing, used to my calling their direct line. I want to let myself go, yelling crazily into my office phone, but I don't. I laugh back and replace the receiver.

Then, suddenly, there it is. The MRI is done. I scrolled through the images. First quickly, then slower. Then a different set of slices from an alternate angle, then another just to make sure. Much slower, taking it all in.

It's clean.

All of the cavernomas were gone, including the one we went back for.

I sat back in my chair and closed my eyes. The wash of relief came over me quickly. I could feel the gratitude suffuse my whole being, rising, then holding for a moment before ebbing. Gratitude that we were able to do what was intended and that he had woken up after the procedure and was doing well. Gratitude that I would be able to walk over to the ICU and let Hayden's family know that his next decade and beyond would be different from his last. It would bring new challenges of course, but those challenges didn't involve the background concern of what that previously present cavernoma would do next year, or the lingering possibility of brain surgery yet again, or the chance that somehow something would happen, a bleed or a slip in the OR, that would forever alter the person you are or how you move through the world around you. There would still be years of follow-up imaging to check, just in case, but the years of deep worry, the time of convincing themselves that all *might* be okay, were done.

Of course, my RTOR rate would now go up, as would yet another metric, LOS—average length of stay—both thought by hospital administration to represent my surgical effectiveness and efficiency. I winced because somehow even after all the years of knowing what was truly important and what was not, I found myself unable to fully let that metric go.

I closed the imaging desktop on my computer, leaned back, and imagined a scene that Hayden had described to me days before, right after that conversation when he learned his cavernoma had grown. It was what he wanted to get back to one day. I could see him straddling the roof of a home he had helped to build. The blue sky overhead, the sound of the nail guns cracking around him. I found myself thinking about the people who would one day live in the homes he built, the lives they would lead. House after house, row after row, subdivision by subdivision, all there because of the miracle of human coordination. And the work of Hayden's hands, now steady, with not a trace of tremor. In that moment in my office, with my eyes closed and thinking of those rows of homes and all those people in them, I reminded myself yet again what was truly important, and all the metrics and self-criticism that could fill my day faded away.

23

The Whole Miracle

SEVERAL YEARS AGO, I was called by a longtime mentor and friend in Utah. His team had pieced back together an eight-year-old boy after a space heater he and his father were huddled around in their garage one cold night exploded. A hunk of hot shrapnel had torn into the right side of the boy's neck, ripped open a hole in the carotid artery, completely severed his jugular vein, damaged other blood vessels, and wreaked havoc on critical nerves. He would have bled out but for the fact that his father held pressure on his neck for hours—first, for the hectic, snowy ride on the drive to the outside hospital, then throughout the ground transfer to the regional children's hospital, and finally right there in the trauma bay until my friend's team took over and got him up to the operating room to repair the damaged blood vessels.

The nerve injury was the reason for the call. Now, months later, the boy had persistent arm weakness; in fact, while some feeling had returned, his right arm was mostly useless. In the operating room that night the Utah team had observed damage to the brachial plexus, a highly intricate webbing of nerves that pass through the area behind the collarbone on their way from the spinal cord to the muscles of the arm.

The brachial plexus is a complex structure that has fascinated me from my earliest days as a medical student as I toiled in the gross

anatomy cadaver lab. From the spinal cord, which runs the length
of the torso, come tiny nerve roots, microscopic at first, that bunch
together and travel through small holes, or nerve foramina, in the
side of the spinal canal. In the cervical spine, the roots enter the shelter of the lateral neck muscles, weave around several critical blood
vessels to and from the head, and begin to converge and divide in a
highly predictable pattern until they emerge under the collarbone
as the five main nerve trunks that innervate the muscles of the arm.
It's fascinating to me because the pattern is, with rare exception, the
same from person to person. The same pattern I saw nearly three
decades ago in cadavers is precisely mirrored in the smaller version
I see in the operating room now as I perform a repair on infants following a particularly traumatic birth. Each time I expose it in the
OR, its form taking shape in front of me as we carefully separate
the surrounding tissue away from the pearly white nerves, I am
reminded of macramé. Beautiful, intricately woven, and fragile.

I met the boy, Leonard, and his father in my clinic a few weeks
after the call. It had been almost six months since the incident. They
sat close, the boy initially burying his face into his father's side. The
dad explained to me how Leonard recovered after the initial lifesaving surgery but that his arm remained paralyzed, completely limp
by his side. Then, around month three, he began to move his wrist
and fingers, a sign that the very longest nerves had recovered. But
that also meant that the nerves that travel the shortest distance, to
the deltoid, the largest shoulder muscle, were not recovering. He
could not move his arm away from his body. Nor were the nerves
that go to the biceps working, which meant that he was incapable
of bending his elbow to, say, bring his hand to his mouth. By four
months after the injury, he had a hand that was gaining strength by
the day, but no way for it to be truly functional. That he'd survived
was a miracle. And the fact that he was going to be able to go to
school and live a full life was equally miraculous.

But what we were there talking about was the possibility of his getting an entirely functioning arm back. I sat with Leonard and his father and discussed surgery, the rationale and also the risk. We would avoid the area of injury entirely. Too much scar and damage, I told them. The risk of injuring that repaired carotid was too high. We would find the nerves down in the arm and do our work there. They listened intently. When I was done, a few moments passed. The father turned to his son, all of eight years old, but who had lived the trauma of years in a few short months.

"What do you want to do, son?" he asked. "It's your arm."

The boy looked up at his father's face. He reached around with his left hand and picked up his own right hand. He wrapped it around his father's neck and then came around the other side with the left one to embrace him. He laid his head on his father's shoulder and whispered an answer, quiet enough just for his father to hear, who then looked up directly at me.

"We want the whole miracle, Doc."

MY FATHER FIRST mentioned his own hand weakness on the day that I asked him to be the best man at my wedding.

Within weeks, he was given his diagnosis of ALS, amyotrophic lateral sclerosis, and regardless of the prodigious amount of reading I did desperately searching for an alternative diagnosis, none of it ever made a difference. Over the next six months, as I finished medical school, the disease progressed relentlessly, as ALS typically does. During those months, I spent more time with him than at any other in my adult life—making the ninety-minute drive back to southern Mississippi from Jackson as often as possible, knowing that soon I would be leaving medical school for residency at Duke and that his decline was inexorable.

I flew next to him as he piloted his plane a few times more in this period, now realizing how I had taken all those years in the sky with him for granted. The last time we flew together was, I believe, his last as a pilot. His hands were visibly weaker. He asked me to reach over and push the throttle in just a bit to slow the plane for the approach. For all the years I had flown with him, I had noticed that each time he landed, he seemed to aim for a spot right on top of the white lines of the runway number. Right at the flare, when the ground comes up and the plane floats down to the tarmac as the airspeed drops, he would just slightly wiggle the yoke. He told me once that it was to ensure the controls were free, but I always saw it as his way of saying to himself that he had successfully made it home, had nailed it on the numbers, yet again.

Once he told me that as the commander of the Air National Guard base in Meridian, he was flying his F-4 Phantom over the Gulf of Mexico and was ahead of schedule. Down beneath him was a navy aircraft carrier. Everyone knows of the competitive spirit that exists between air force and navy pilots. The navy always maintained that they were the better pilots because of the simple fact that they landed *their* jets on carriers, sometimes at night. The air force thought this was ridiculous, of course. Up there that day at seventy-five hundred feet in a clear sky, ahead of schedule, my father saw an opportunity and took it. He requested an approach to the carrier. Not a full landing, but just an approach where he would come around at just enough distance and altitude to see what the deck looked like rolling up and down in the whitecaps.

He recounted this story to me on a flight to Miami during those magical six months when we spent as much time together as possible, both of us knowing that I was leaving and he was dying. I asked him if he'd had some epiphany after he had made that approach on the carrier.

"Son, I looked at that tiny deck pitching up and down in the water, and I did realize something," he said. "Those navy boys may not be the best pilots at flying, but damn if they may be the best ones at *landing.*"

That flight to Miami was so that my father could participate in an ongoing phase 3 clinical trial at the University of Miami looking at the effect of a particular neurotrophic factor on life expectancy and quality of life in patients with ALS. When we arrived, the walk from the gate to the baggage belt was longer than he anticipated, and I called for a wheelchair that he was not ready to admit that he needed. My eldest sister, who lived near Miami, met us in an open-top Jeep, and Dad's arms were so weak from the disease that on the ride he was unable to wipe sweat away or brush his hair aside as the wind blew it into his face.

Within a few minutes of arrival at the clinic, he received an intravenous injection of the study drug, which was followed by a series of strength tests that only highlighted how weak the once-strongest man in my life had become. Years later, after he died, we found out that the drug was actually the placebo and not the study drug—but it made no actual difference, as it turned out, because the study drug was found to be ineffectual.

The taxi ride back to the airport was delayed by heavy traffic. I hastily rolled him to the gate, and we were just late enough that they had stopped loading passengers. In those days, the gate door was left unlocked while last-minute adjustments were being made. Despite the warning signs, Dad instructed me to push him past the gate agent counting the boarding passes and through the door. A claxon sounded. Several agents quickly descended upon us.

"Keep rolling," he said. I set my vision forward. There was a jolt. We kept moving. We came to the end of the Jetway. A two-foot-wide gap had opened up because the jet bridge had been pulled back in preparation for the flight taxiing out of the gate. The heat of the late day curled in around the opening between the jet bridge and the fuselage.

The pilot looked over through the cockpit side window, surprised. The three visibly angry agents around us yelled over the engines and motioned with their arms for us to come away from the edge. One picked up the phone at the end of the jet bridge to call for emergency help.

My father tried to raise his arm, his limp hand dangling, and was just able to motion for the pilot to open up the sliding window. Despite the gap, the flight deck was only a few feet away. There was chaos all around us. I had no idea how I would explain this to the dean of my medical school.

"I'm Colonel John Wellons, retired commander of the 186th Air National Guard wing," my father somehow shouted through the noise. "Served for over forty years. I have ALS, am in an experimental trial at the University of Miami, and my son is trying to get me home. He's in medical school. We're late because of traffic and I am sorry for it. Can you get us home, Captain?"

The pilot looked at my dad, then at me, then back at him again. He leaned back in the cockpit and spoke into the radio microphone, looked back out at the agents, and nodded.

The pilot motioned for one of the agents to extend the Jetway closer. The agents waved off the arriving emergency help. We moved away from the edge as the two-foot gap disappeared. Soon the aircraft door opened, and two female flight attendants looked out dumbfounded at the five of us there.

"Well, don't just wait here, Jay," Dad whispered to me through the corner of his mouth. "Get us in there!"

We got the wheelchair through the door and onto the flight. Dad, tired from the exertion, needed more help than normal getting into his seat on the aisle. The agents kindly took the chair off the plane, turning back to wave at my father as they left. He mustered a warm smile back.

The cockpit door opened. Soon the pilot appeared in front of us.

"Well, I figured it must have been air force brass causing all this ruckus," he said, a broad smile spreading across his face. He introduced himself. "Retired navy myself, Colonel," he said. "Made it to captain before taking it to civilian life, mostly for the wife."

"Captain," my dad replied, "I cannot thank you enough."

"You are welcome, Colonel. My pleasure. Now you sit back,

relax, and know this flight is brought to you courtesy of the U.S. Navy," he said, smiling. With a quick salute, he was gone.

I sat in stunned silence as the engine whine picked up and we continued our taxi. The other passengers quietly stole glances in our direction, then looked back down at their reading as all returned to normal.

"Well," my dad quietly said, turning his head to mine and smiling, "at least we know we're in for a good landing."

THE BOY FROM Utah lay asleep on the OR table, his entire right arm, neck, and chest prepped out in a ritual elaborate enough that my partners compare it to my draping an altar for worship. The arm is up away from the body at a ninety-degree angle and rotated into a waving position, the hand lying back on a pile of four folded towels. Today, we are going for the miracle. But we are not stupid. We are not going back into the explosion site on the side of the neck with its jagged scar and risk of opening up the repaired vessels. Our plan today is to rob from Peter to pay Paul—to find nerves farther down in the arm that have extra innervation, or input, to their target muscles and use those spare nerve bundles to reinnervate the nonfunctioning muscles.

The rhythmic hiss of the ventilator comes from around the drapes. We've carefully exposed several of the nerves within the cleft, through an incision that runs along the deep groove between the biceps and the triceps muscles along the inner upper arm. The operating microscope is brought into the field once we find our targets: the wispy nerve going directly into the biceps muscle and the ulnar nerve, whose primary function is to flex the wrist and fingers. Under the scope, we open up the epineurium of the ulnar nerve, the protective sheath that must be cut lengthwise to expose the tiny and fragile smaller nerve bundles—the fascicles—inside. The technician sitting at the nerve-monitoring console warns us that we've irritated the nerve slightly, as expected, but no damage.

Before each case like this—once we've prepped but before we make the skin incision—I carefully place tiny pairs of needles through the skin in the major muscles of the arm and hand. The needles are attached to multicolored wires that trail down the arm and run down the side of the OR table across the length of the room to a monitoring station, manned by a technician specially trained just for these cases. By monitoring the status of the muscles, he can give us a road map and update on the nerves that we are interested in, all registering as rows and rows of squiggly lines on a screen. This monitoring is extremely helpful when performing complex nerve surgery, and today it is key: We are going to do more than irritate the nerve. We are going to cut it, at least part of it, so we will need to be damn sure about what part not to cut before we do. We press on.

For this part of the operation, we have to find the nerve fascicle within the ulnar nerve that innervates the muscles that cause wrist flexion. One of the many miracles of the human body is that there are structures here and there that are redundant, like having a spare kidney, or ovary/testicle, or the blood vessels to and from the brain on *both* sides of the neck. Here, we will use this redundancy in something more like a hack. There are several muscles that allow us to flex our wrist, and they are innervated by two main nerves, the ulnar nerve and the median nerve. Our plan for this first part of the operation is to find that redundant input that runs in the tiny fascicles of the ulnar nerve, cut them, and then use them to help regain the function in the biceps by sewing them into the nerve going into the biceps muscle, its function lost upstream when the plexus was damaged. Over time, as the nerve heals, the brain retrains the nerve to do an entirely different action than initially intended. Hence, the hack.

We dissect out the ulnar nerve fascicles. The operating microscope is at as high a magnification as possible, a tiny beam of light illuminates our work in the otherwise darkened OR. We use a hook-shaped probe to stimulate our target. Once we confirm the correct fascicle, we cut it.

I hear a slight yelp from the corner of the room.

"Hey, Doc, something just happened. Not good," said the tech, anxiously.

"Ah, sorry," I said. I had forgotten to tell him we were about to cut it. "All good, we're about to start one of the repairs," I respond.

"Chest pain, Doc," he replies. "You know you give me chest pain when you do that."

I smile under my mask and continue. Using tiny scissors, we then cut the nerve going into the biceps, making sure both the ulnar fascicle and the target nerve have enough length on them to connect. Then we sew the two nerves together. It's so tiny that any unintended air current in the room can blow the suture out from under the microscope and right out of our view. Oftentimes, I have to remind myself to breathe when I do this work as I try to keep the rest of my body as still as possible. The proximal end of the usable fascicle from the ulnar nerve is sutured into the distal end of the nerve stump going into the muscle, the ends connected in a way to help guide the individual nerve growths across the microscopic gap.

"Looks good from the cheap seats," the scrub nurse says, seeing all of this play out on the video screen in front of her.

"We're halfway done," I say. "Next up, the armpit." Now we need to work on restoring his shoulder movement. We extend our incision deep into the boy's cleaned and exposed right axilla, the medical term for the armpit. Our target is the rich network of blood vessels and nerves just underneath its thin skin. We are working closer to the damage this time, farther up the brachial plexus, but coming up just beneath the injured area. Soon we find our two intended nerves, stimulate them, and prepare for the second part of the operation. This procedure, like the one just done, is called a neurotization, or nerve transfer, and is a technique whose origins, yet again, lay in the lessons learned from the surgeons and soldiers in World War I, now more than a century ago.

The triceps muscle in the back of our upper arm has three heads, hence the "tri-" of triceps. And each muscle head has its own nerve branch going to it that comes from the radial nerve. Leonard's triceps, unlike the biceps and deltoid, happens to have regained full function over time, he can straighten his arm fine. So here comes our hack again. This muscle works just fine with only two heads intact, so one branch can be rerouted. The long branch is cut (this time remembering to warn our technician). We swing it way up to the axillary nerve that goes to the large deltoid muscle, deep in the axilla, that is responsible for most arm movement at the shoulder. We then cut the axillary nerve and proceed to make our microscopic repair. Once finished, we swiftly make our way out, closing up muscle layers and skin until we are done.

As neurosurgeons, oftentimes we refer to our work with cerebrospinal fluid as "just like plumbing" and with nerves as "like being an electrician." But in truth, just like in the previous story, repairing nerves is not like splicing wire ends together, after which, with a click of the switch, the light comes on. The effect is far from immediate. The nerve grows back slowly, one millimeter a day at best. This result is as if the electrician leaves your home, rugs unrolled into place, furniture scooted back, bill paid, but the lights don't switch on for six to nine months. Each time we do this, no matter how much warning up front, it feels like years pass in the interval.

Six months later, I saw the father and son in the same clinic room where I first met them. They were both radiant.

"He can't wait to show you," said his dad.

"Well, show me!" I said to the boy. "I can't wait either!"

He picked up the left arm and waved.

"The *right* arm, Leonard!" I said, and we all laughed.

There are discussions that you have with patients before surgery. Honest ones. Deeply honest, in which parents and often the children hear about why surgery is needed. Sometimes it's obvious; sometimes it's risky. But there is never, ever, a guarantee. No guarantee that it will work as intended, and no guarantee that there won't be a complication of surgery. In the field of pediatric neurosurgery outside the brain, like in the spine or brachial plexus, there is always a blood vessel nearby, or a nerve, or the spinal cord itself. In the intracranial work that we do, the ability to speak or move or see can be millimeters away. I feel it is my responsibility to ensure that folks understand the risks of surgery and temper the expectations. Probably instilled in me by mentor Jerry Oakes, who once was told by the nurses at Great Ormond Street Hospital for Children in London to quit talking to the families before surgery because he "was frightening the patients with all the dithering on about possible complications."

In the discussion that occurred before this surgery, in this very room, I had told them that we would be happy if he regained the ability to touch his nose and move his arm several degrees away from his body out to the side. What Leonard did instead was hold both arms up signaling a touchdown. We all loudly hooted. The resident and nurse looked in on us from out in the clinic hall to see all three of us in a joyous embrace.

Then Leonard looked at me. "One more thing, Dr. Wellons," he said, and brought his right arm up to his forehead and saluted.

It's a simple gesture, one that happens every day. But whenever I see it, no matter where I am, I see my father. Leonard had no way to know this as we all celebrated his recovery there in that exam room. In truth, not only do I see my father, but I see both him and me, as versions from our past. Me as a two-year-old in the photograph that sat on the veneered side table next to the den couch in my childhood home. A photograph I saw every day growing up. Serious. Son of a military pilot. Saluting directly into the camera. I see my father walking toward me as I waited just off one of the many taxiways from our past, a smile on his face, returning my salute as he leans toward me. I see that last trip we took together on the flight back from Miami. The kind airline pilot honoring him. My father's resolute face looking back, no longer able to bring his hand up to his head, but the intention there as if he had. I think back to how, when he was alive, my father had no idea where exactly my path would lead. To this life, to all these patients, to this very boy. This one salute. I could feel Leonard's gesture pass through me, back through time and space and memory to my father. And I saw him striding toward us all in that clinic room gathered around that exam table, looking toward us, smiling, and saluting back. Father and son and father and son.

Epilogue

———•———

Millimeters and Trajectories

THE NEUROSURGERY RESIDENTS here at our medical center meet for Journal Club every Tuesday evening like clockwork. During it, they discuss topics spanning a wide range of our field: from a meticulous review of detailed internal brainstem anatomy to the stepwise discussion of surgical approaches to complex skull base tumors, from a recent groundbreaking paper published in the *Journal of Neurosurgery* to hands-on training on the application of a halo vest for cervical spine fractures. Both high science and practical learning.

There is also food.

Each time, without fail, food. It is the very least we can do for the work they do. A well-known tenet of neurosurgical training (due to the unpredictability of the schedule and long hours) is to *Eat when you can, sleep when you can, and don't #%^& with the hypothalamus* (general surgeons say "pancreas" there). Hence every Tuesday night they gather for food and for learning.

But the truth of it is that it is mostly just for the opportunity to be with *someone else whose day was like the one I just had,* to do their best to try to process the intensity of it all. It is not easy in the trenches of neurosurgery training.

On this Tuesday night, however, instead of a sterile hospital conference room with the blinds pulled down and the hum of the projector, ten of them sit around the back porch of my house in a wide circle of white chairs. Each of us in blue scrubs and tired from the workday. Plates full of food are casually balanced on knees, half-drained cans of craft beer sit nearby on the floor. The residents who are still operating or dealing with emergencies aren't here, but it is a terrific showing nonetheless. On the theory that telling stories about the things that most affect us is a redemptive act and will help us all—patient and practitioner—in the push to heal, I've asked them to talk about a case that taught them something or that stays with them, or perhaps even haunts them. This is our very first group foray into something like this, formally called narrative medicine, and I admit concern that they would have found reasons not to come that sounded legitimate—*Sorry boss, need to check on a patient one more time* or *Big case tomorrow, need to prepare*—and we would have ended up with three of them at most, tentatively told narratives, and little discussion (and lots of leftover shish kebabs). But thankfully, that is not the case. After the publication of a couple of essays that I had written, a few of the residents mentioned to me that they had some experiences of their own they wished to share with one another and would that be possible?

As the evening wore on and we quieted into the communal telling, some recounted stories of saves or averted disasters they were particularly proud of. Of people who walked away alive because of an unheralded act, large or small, the resident had done, or a complex problem solved. Others admitted to deep losses, telling stories of someone's loved one gone forever, and that inescapable early guilt that comes with feeling like you did not work hard enough or were not smart enough to fix the problem, when most often there simply was nothing to be done.

As I said, this life is not easy.

Medicine is full of stories. Dramatic stories. Hang around a hospital long enough and you will see that these stories need no embellishment. And in neurosurgery, these stories tend to be even more dramatic. They are often the stories at the junction of life and death, of suffering and of joy, of profound spiritual crisis and just-answered prayers. It is impossible to keep from being drawn into these elemental moments when life feels at its most precious and meaningful. Living in this space tends to heighten everything. The embrace of loved ones lasts just a bit longer than before. The breaths in and out while on a hike in nature are a touch deeper. The gratitude for safety and health comes closer to the surface now.

COVID-19 brought much of medicine closer to this place.

I've mostly tried to stay away from the topic of COVID-19 while writing this book. The stories of this pandemic belong to the people sickened by the virus, or the family members left behind or there to pick up the pieces. It also belongs to those individuals courageous and dedicated enough to man the front lines in order to care for them. In the years to come, as we reckon with the virus as a public health calamity and historical event, there will be many more such stories.

One surgical experience during the crisis does stand out to me, though. It was soon after the vaccine was rolled out to healthcare workers across the country, and was the first time that it felt as if we would one day be past all of this. When normal came back to visit for just a moment.

One evening, during the snowstorm that blanketed most of the South in February 2021, our on-call team was rushing to get the operating room ready for an emergency craniotomy on a ten-year-old boy with an epidural hematoma, a life-threatening blood clot between the skull and the covering of the brain. He had been sledding with his friends down an icy hill in his neighborhood as twilight turned to dark. The boy's final attempt shot him out so fast and so far that he slid into the icy street and under a car parked on the other side. Because his head was up trying to see where he was going, he hit the lower door frame, and hard. He turned his head just in time so that the left side took the brunt of the impact instead of his face.

At the scene, he was briefly unconscious but quickly came around. When the EMTs arrived to take him to the local hospital, he was talking easily and showing no signs of confusion, only a headache from where he hit the door frame. The initial brain CT was reassuring but still concerning, showing a small fracture and the tiny epidural hematoma. By the time he was transferred to us for observation, he had become much worse, the clot had expanded substantially and the pressure on the brain was obvious. He lapsed into unconsciousness. Without surgery, he would die.

The door to the OR banged open. It was the circulating nurse who had gone with the anesthesia team and my resident to get the patient.

"Hey, guys," she said. "We have an issue."

We all looked up: the scrub nurse, the resident who had come in and was now pulling up the films, the nurse anesthetist, and me.

What now? I thought.

"The rapid COVID test isn't back yet."

Remember, this was after we had figured out how to diagnose the virus quickly and consistently, and the vaccine had just been made available to the elderly and those in healthcare. In the days before that, each time we did an emergency operation without knowing the patient's COVID-19 status, we used adequate PPE and took the necessary precautions. Still, the idea that you were making a potentially life-threatening decision every time you went to the OR for a trauma case was always there. At the start of the year, *Forbes* reported that nearly 300,000 healthcare workers had contracted COVID-19 and somewhere between 900 and 1,700 had died. Most of those healthcare workers were in emergency departments and ICUs, but it was difficult not to feel as if you were destined to be the next statistic.

This time, however, for the first time in a year, things were different.

"You guys all vaccinated?" I asked.

"Yes," came the answer from everyone in the room.

"Well, let's get going then," the scrub nurse cut in and said. "We've got work to do."

Soon we were all moving through the familiar pace of surgery, of doing our jobs in the middle of the night. In the early morning hours when we were done, when typically we'd move in our own directions to try to steal some sleep before rounds or prepare the OR for the next day, we all waited and watched as the anesthesiologist took out the boy's breathing tube. We smiled under our masks as he held up three fingers on each hand and wiggled his toes to command. For that moment, as we all hovered over this one boy's bed and shook hands, all was right in the world again.

BUT THE WORLD will not be made right so easily.

Because, of course, COVID, and the COVID vaccine and even basic public health measures, would cause a profound rupture in our society. Between science and its opposite. Reason and unreason. Cities and small towns. And in a deeply personal way, between my past and my present. Just as the neurosurgery residents who gathered for Journal Club had something they needed to share so as not to carry the burden alone, so, too, do I. As I end this book, and take the measure of all that I have learned, this is the story that remains heaviest on my heart.

Several weeks before writing this, I watched on the news as a local school board meeting near Nashville devolved into chaos. Healthcare workers were shouted down and followed out to their cars. A pediatric intensive care doctor responsible for saving hundreds of children's lives over her years here, who had attended in order to speak in favor of school mask mandates, was threatened by fist-shaking agitators surrounding her car.

We know where you live! We will find you!

As both the pandemic and the politics rage, these attitudes seem particularly concentrated in the South, the land where I was born and raised and where I live still. As of this writing, my home state of Mississippi ranked near the bottom in vaccinations against the deadly virus. I look around the current landscape in my current home of Tennessee and recognize the dissenters. They look a great deal like people I took care of and knew in Alabama, where I spent my first ten years in practice, or North Carolina, where I trained, or in my small hometown of Columbia, Mississippi. They are people who look a lot like me from a demographic perspective: white, southern, and Christian. Many are like the folks I played with in the backyards of my childhood, went to elementary school classes and middle school dances with. They are very much like the people who stacked sandbags along with my family to protect our historic downtown whenever the Pearl River would flood, who brought food when my grandmother was sick, who came to both of my parents' funerals, and who loved our whole family through loss and triumph. And whom we in turn, then and now, love back.

I was born into this and grew up twenty miles from the north-south Mississippi-Louisiana border. In our sizable, warm, and always well-lit white square-columned home on Main Street lived for many years some combination of my mother, father, two older sisters, and me. As of this writing, Eve, the oldest, lives there with several animals, marking over fifty years that a member of the same Wellons family has lived in it. When visiting in years past and most recently for funerals, my friends have fondly referred to it as the family museum. "Is there a guided tour?" asked one. "Gift shop?"

Soon I will be cleaning it out in preparation for sale, and that feels to me akin to facing a third parent's death. The history of my family, and all of those memories, live on in that place. If, per chance, one would like to see the hand-sewn multicolor butterfly costume my middle sister, Sarah, wore in her school play her sophomore year, it was saved by my mother, hung in plastic wrap in the orderly attic, with the antennae headband looped around the hanger. Curious about any awards that I won in my years of middle school science fair enthusiasm? Those ribbons are immortalized on the wall of the room that I grew up in. The same room, I might add, in which my father spent his final weeks until his last trip to the hospital. The very same room where my mother died twenty years later, surrounded by her family. Yes, the room that I lived in as a child is the same room that both of my parents lay dying in. So please, give me a pass if I have to triple my therapy visits as the time comes to let that house go. It will not be easy.

Both sisters were out of the house by the time I was in junior high, so I lived first as the youngest of three, then of two, and finally as an only child. We were a family who loved one another the best we knew how. We went to the local Episcopal church with sixteen members as opposed to those with hundreds in the other faith communities in the area. (The only other child in the church and I both took Sunday school classes with the adults. He and I knew the word "eschatology" by the sixth grade.) Our family took vacations together when possible, ate our meals around the dining room table at night, and were full of imperfections and issues that we had only a vague idea of at the time. In those early years, we made homecoming floats for my sisters in the garage, had a sister's occasional boyfriend show up on a motorcycle, and endured just enough tragedy to keep us aware that life was fragile and to soldier on.

That is who I was and am. But I am someone else now, too. And as such I stand astride two worlds—my small Mississippi town and a world-class medical center at Vanderbilt University in Nashville. Being inside the world of science, I cannot help having evolved over my life: scientifically, culturally, and religiously. And this is certainly not just my story. It is the story of many of us in the world today, in medicine or not. Formed by our family and place of origin, shaped by our life experiences, sloughing off superstitions, embracing proof alongside faith, and now in positions to effect change in our society.

As the virus was on the march, the mistrust that should have been directed at rampant misinformation and crank science was instead aimed squarely at doctors and nurses and life-saving medical researchers. And much of that rage came from the world I know best. In *You Can't Go Home Again,* the great American writer Thomas Wolfe, a North Carolina boy, told the story of a writer who, in a hit novel, depicts his town in a way that makes his neighbors furious. Hence the title. But Wolfe also meant that one can't seek refuge in the past: "You can't go . . . back home to the old forms and systems of things which once seemed everlasting but which are changing all the time—back home to the escapes of Time and Memory."

If there has ever been a challenge to the escapes of Time and Memory, it is science. Science obeys its own schedule, and does not observe the vagaries of elections, news cycles, cultural proclivities, or the burdens of history. For truly valid research to look at both outcomes and complications in a rigorous fashion, time must pass in order to determine the best evidence for a particular intervention or disprove the same. We have become used to answers that come in the same way that all information is delivered now: in 24/7 sound bites where the positioning of the story is determined by the number of clicks rather than its truth or actual value to society. Of course, immediate results and corner-cutting are not how conducting reasonable research works, at least the kind of research that does not result in false or even harmful recommendations.

The initial association of child vaccination with autism, now debunked, is worth examining. A small study published in 1998 in *The Lancet,* a well-respected medical journal, revealed an unexpected association between childhood vaccinations and autism in eight out of twelve patients. No causation was ever proven, the paper was observational only. The result of this small study was the

near-derailing of a vaccination program for children that had func-
tionally eradicated measles, mumps, rubella, and other childhood
diseases that had previously greatly impacted society. Pediatricians,
used to automatically vaccinating children, now had hard push-back.
The great irony, when compared to the present day, is that this was
typically from parents more liberal in their political leanings. Yes,
vaccination hesitancy back then was specific to mostly left-of-center
young parents who fell victim to the hyper-media of the time, the
individual stories of parents looking for a reason their child was
autistic, and the resonance of a myth repeated again and again over
the years. Twelve years later, the author of the initial paper was
found to have fabricated the data. It was completely made-up. The
entire paper was a lie. *The Lancet* published a full retraction, yet the
damage had been done. And we are reckoning with that damage to
this day.

Maybe I'm like Thomas Wolfe's protagonist and can't go home
again. But then, I never left. By grace, a lot of luck, and good parents and friends, I have been privileged to make the journeys with
patients that are recorded in this book right here in the South—
a short drive but a world away from where I was born and raised.
One day, the pandemic will be but a memory. But we will be left with
the residual effect on our culture, in particular the often withering
judgment leveled at those whom we see as not like us. For our own
good, we must make that cultural chasm a memory, too. By forgetting the anger. By remembering that we are more alike than we
are different, no matter what point on the compass you call home.
That our origins are often so very similar, set apart by only millimeters and trajectories, before life took us far away from one another.
We must remember that forgiveness is an important part of human
relationships. We are all capable of the grace and resilience shown
by the children and their parents in these pages. That is one of the
main reasons why I decided to write this book—because reaching
out to one another with an open hand, and sharing stories from the

depths of our lives, of our joys as well as our pain, is the best way to remember that we are all human, that none of us is born lesser or estranged or alien, and that we all face the same essential and imponderable bare facts of existence. Talking to one another—and telling our stories, communicating across divides—just might be our salvation. I believe that the stories of these families and others like them will be critical as we help one another toward healing.

BY THE END of Journal Club that evening at my house, the paper plates were stuffed into the compost bin and the food was packed up to take to the residents on call at the hospital. All of the residents in attendance had spoken but one. I had led the discussions a bit but mostly sat back and listened to them all talk and process. One resident had spoken of an elderly woman that she had admitted from the ED and connected with, "country strong" as she described her. She was diagnosed with a malignant brain tumor and underwent resection, but her ultimate and too-early death had left this resident with significant grief. "How did she go from country strong to barely alive? What else could we have done?" she asked. "Why are we still so far from a cure?"

The last resident to speak sheepishly admitted that he had not written anything down but would it be okay if he told us his story? He proceeded to tell us of a young man in his mid-twenties who had made it to the ED barely alive. His basilar artery, the main artery supplying blood to the brainstem, had clotted off. The ensuing stroke that was happening before this resident's eyes looked like it was going to be devastating. People typically do not recover from this. Oftentimes they are locked in—aware of their surroundings but unable to move or communicate. This resident, at the time beginning to develop an interest in endovascular techniques—like those mentioned in "Rupture"—was able to get the patient up to the angiogram suite quickly, and he and the attending promptly opened up the blood vessel. "It was miraculous," he said.

Then the resident's voice quavered, ever so slightly. "Post-op, he woke up," he said, pausing for a moment. "A complete recovery." He took his gaze just above and past us, as if he could see another reality playing out behind us. He looked back and refocused. "I know this is what I want to do now," he said. Then he sat back down and we were done.

What was clear to me was that these young doctors *needed* to tell their stories to one another. To process the significance of what they were doing every day, to reckon with the feelings that they were coming home with every night. There were no easy answers. But the residents spoke of their patients with such empathy, such immense respect. They remembered their courage in the face of the unknown as they rolled them back to the operating room or watched them wake up in the ICU after surgery. These collective memories seemed to help us all immeasurably as we grappled with things too big for any one person to bear alone.

In neurosurgery, we walk with our patients and learn profound lessons from them along the way. But the realization that we are fragile, that our lives can turn in a moment, is a constant for all of us, regardless of our path in life. Understanding that we and those we love are not immune to pain and suffering is only one feature of our covenant here on earth. Redemption from that fear comes in the awe-inspiring capacity for resilience, grace, and healing that we possess—for evidence of this, look no further than the children in these pages.

I'm honored to be a part of these stories and grateful for the precious lives behind them, for these residents, colleagues, and other co-workers inside neurosurgery and out who keep me grounded and offer me invaluable perspective. I have been blessed by the opportunity to pass along a part of the lives of these remarkable children and their parents. And to tell something of the story of how in this life we are all both the healers and the healed.

Acknowledgments

———•———

THERE ARE SO many people to thank that I could easily make this the longest part of the entire book. After fifty-two years on this earth and half of it in the world of medicine, neurosurgery, and pediatric neurosurgery, I have a great many people to whom I am indebted for help and influence along the way. If I have inadvertently left you off this list, please forgive me.

First and foremost, to the children and parents whose journeys you have allowed me to be a part of, thank you. Uniformly, you were all supportive of this effort and that was critical to me from the outset. I dearly hope that this book helps you all to understand that it has been my honor to care for you and your children, and that in the midst of your own healing, I have in many ways been healed too. The gratitude that you have offered me so kindly goes both ways, equally.

Thank you to my most wonderful spouse of over twenty-five years, Melissa, who has been a part of my life on and off since middle school. You are my greatest earthly treasure and I love you dearly. To my children, Jack and Fair, who have endured my early-morning and weekend writing and (occasional) grumpiness at burning the entire candle at once, I love you both very much. I am so very grateful that you are both in our lives. Now please clean up your room and feed the dog.

When I was recovering from surgery back in 2017 and was on forced bedrest for most of the fall, it was my sister Sarah Laird Kochey who encouraged me to "start jotting some of those stories from work down" and who first had the belief in me that I could one day become a writer. What a powerful force for good in this life you are, Sarah. Thank you. I am grateful to Trish Hall for her immensely important early advice and editing prowess and the phenomenal editor Peter Catapano at *The New York Times* for taking a chance on an unpublished pediatric neurosurgeon who had encountered a profuse nosebleed on a flight to Vermont.

From that and the next *Times* essay, came my agent, David Granger of Aevitas Creative Management, a force multiplier in my life, whose fascinating life journey should also one day be chronicled. His initial request to me was to "let it flow" and write out five thousand words stream-of-consciousness style on the path I took into pediatric neurosurgery. That over time took shape as the Introduction of a formal book proposal, and ultimately the Prologue to *All That Moves Us*. The very initial version, sans punctuation, capitalization, and correct spelling, reads more like a caffeine- and sleep-deficit-induced vision quest falling far short of my James Joyce–ian aspirations and remains safely ensconced in a protected hard drive the whereabouts of which are known only to me.

At that point, Mark Warren and Penguin Random House formally entered the picture. A tremendous thank-you to Nancy Jo Iacoi for her role in connecting sister Sarah and Mark in the early days of this journey. I cannot begin to thank Mark enough for being my editor. My last published nonscientific work up until 2019 was . . . never, and working with him has been a master class in writing and editing. Over the course of constructing this book, Mark has been a patient and gifted teacher. I am beyond grateful for his ability to pull out of me more than just narrative but also the words that these children and families deserve. In the process, not only did I become a better writer, but my ability to look back over these experiences and glean the meaning from them as they apply to my own life deepened profoundly. Thank you, Mark. There is a whole team from Penguin Random House to thank, and this includes publisher

Andy Ward, deputy publisher Tom Perry, assistant editor Chayenne Skeete, Rachel Ake for her beautiful cover design, the marketing team of Ayelet Durantt, Barbara Fillon, and Emani Glee and publicity director London King for their terrific ideas and absolute devotion to this book, and our production editor Mark Birkey, for the great care he took with every sentence.

I have several friends to thank specific to this book: Abhaya Kulkarni for reading over the entire manuscript, helping to bind it tighter before I sent it to PRH; Jon Meacham for his influence and insight into the publishing world; Brad and Kimberly Williams Paisley for reminding me of the immense importance of creativity in our lives; Reed Omary for our morning walks; Cal Turner, Jr., for the lunches and past stories of my family; Jamie Kyne for his calming words; Jerry Martin for his lawyer recommendations and enthusiasm—and John Voigt and Kim Schefler for said lawyering; Catherine Seltzer and Amanda Little for key writing advice in the final hours; Allen Sills for his incredibly effective devil's advocacy; Ash Shah for quickly accepting the new guy from Mississippi in our early years together as interns at Duke; and Reid Thompson—friend, chairman, and gifted surgeon—for his unwavering support of me over the years.

In addition to those noted in the Prologue, it is critical to recognize the role of three professors in the department of English at the University of Mississippi in the late 1980s who supported me, early on as a student of literature, and later into my life in medicine: Chris Fitter, now professor at Rutgers University; Colby Kullman, professor emeritus at the University of Mississippi; and Gregory Schirmer, also professor and chair emeritus at the University of Mississippi. In order, one connected me to Shakespeare, one to Swift, and one to Joyce and Yeats. For these lifelong gifts I will be forever grateful. Dr. Fitter, you were right. There is always an applicable Shakespeare quote, even in the operating room. Perhaps especially in the operating room.

To the residents and fellows I have worked with, current as well as over the past two decades, thank you. My career is so much more meaningful for having you there along the way and I cannot conceive of this life in neurosurgery without this aspect of it.

Thank you to the surgeons, medical doctors, and other healthcare personnel at the University of Mississippi Medical Center and Duke University Medical Center who were a part of training me (specifically chairmen Andy Parent at UMMC and Allan Friedman at Duke), to my co-students and residents along the way, and to all the many people in the "bucket line" who put in the time at each stop.

To Jerry Oakes, early fellowship mentor, senior partner at UAB, and friend, none of this entire career happens without your influence. Thank you. Shane Tubbs, a walking *Gray's Anatomy* and Netter's *Atlas* combined, I'm grateful for your early partnership and lifelong friendship. Thank you to my other partners at UAB (Paul Grabb and Jeff Blount, then Leslie Akapo-Satchivi, Curtis Rozzelle, and Jim Johnston) who endured my early years as a driven academic surgeon and who have remained my friends over the years, despite, I am certain, their occasional inclinations otherwise.

To my current pediatric neurosurgery partners at Vanderbilt (Rob Naftel, Chris Bonfield, and Michael Dewan) who have supported this effort from the beginning, thank you. Moreover, thank you for your friendship and wise counsel, and for sharing our connected vision for what we have built in our division together. You are all immensely talented surgeons and deeply good human beings and I am grateful for your influence on me.

To the rest of the faculty and support staff in the departments of neurosurgery at both UAB (in particular, Amy Finch and Nadine Bradley) and Vanderbilt (Pam Lane and business officer Coleman Harris), I am grateful for your help and collegiality over the years as well. Debi Andrews, my administrative wingman (I have no other title that better explains the importance of her role), has been absolutely critical in nearly all endeavors that I have been involved with. You are an enabler in the highest sense—a profound thanks to you as well.

I have been fortunate to have had many bosses who have influenced and supported me along the years. In addition to those already listed, I am particularly grateful to Jim Markert, Luke Gregory (posthumously), Meg Rush, John Brock, Jeff Upperman, and VUMC Chairman of the Section of Surgical Sciences Seth Karp. (Without fail, Seth always finished our meetings with *How's the writing going?*) A special thank-you to Jeff Balser, president of VUMC, who has been supportive of my writing from the very beginning.

To all the scrub techs, circulating nurses, anesthesia personnel, clinic teams, ICU teams, and ward nurses along the way, please know that none of this would have been possible without you. A special thanks to Debbie Carciopolo, Martin Kircus, Maria Sullivan, Diana Penn, Kayla Gross, Melissa Gordon, Jon Kraft, Jason Linsley, Tasha Lewis, and Laura Newsom for such hard work and dedication. And especially to Nick Metoyer for handing me what I needed in the OR instead of what I asked for.

A note on the constant friendship and hard work of Haley Vance, our phenomenal nurse practitioner partner, who has walked much of the journey with these children and me. Her dedication to the families and ability to handle so much of the emotional swings of our practice is Oslerian in its immensity. Chevis Shannon, clinical outcomes researcher and also friend of many years, has had an enormous influence on my ability to see epidemiological problems on a larger scale and has influenced me to formal study resulting in a midlife degree in epidemiology. I am grateful to both of you for these things and much more.

There are so many friends and colleagues throughout the field of pediatric neurosurgery outside of my own practice who have influenced me along the way. Foremost in this group not already mentioned are John Kestle, Jay Riva-Cambrin, Dave Limbrick, and Bill

Whitehead, all colleagues from the formative days of the Hydro-cephalus Clinical Research Network, a clinical research group from which comes I believe our most important research and influence on our field. To my many colleagues in the American Society of Pediatric Neurosurgeons, I am truly grateful. Please know that a great deal of this whole endeavor is in honor of the work that all of you do for children. Thank you to John Jane, Sr. (posthumously), and Jim Rutka, sequential editors-in-chief of the *Journal of Neurosurgery*, for teaching me a great deal about medical writing and editing (and to Jim in particular for his enthusiasm and tolerance for my early nontraditional scientific editorials). To Benny Iskandar, Matt Smyth, and Mark Krieger, you all influence me more than you know, in neurosurgery and in life. Thank you. To Jon Martin, Susan Durham, and Ed Smith, one day we will run that miserable-sounding race together, I promise.

A quick thank-you to Elizabeth and Clark Akers and Carter and Glynn Brazzell for the use of their respective cabins in the woods (and away from the Internet) in the final days of book-writing and editing. And to my cousins Charlie, Will, and Lee Haraway, whose music, including as the Haraway Brothers and the Sundogs, has given me so much joy and inspiration in this process. I firmly believe that everyone should listen to their "Song of Resurrection" at least once in their lives. I am grateful for my cousin Brad Wellons, who has been a lifelong friend and a keeper of family stories, and who walked his own path with his father, Kennard, my father's brother. I would also like to thank sister-in-law Julia Myrick and her husband, Dan, as well as Allen Murphy, Andrew Foxworth, Ollie Rencher, William Henderson, and Joanna Storey—all friends supportive of my creative side. We are fortunate to have so many supportive friends in Nashville, including Keith Meacham, Gray Sasser, Kathryn Sasser, Vandana and Rick Abramson, Amanda and Ben Henley, and Cyndee Martin. Also, and only semi-humorously, to my family's wonderful Cavapoo, Watney, who has slept next to my feet in the last months of writing this book, taken me on walks (or river paddles) when I've needed a break, and who has been a companion and confidant in this and many other things.

As I near the end, I would like to thank my sister Eve, who lives in our hometown of Columbia, Mississippi, for keeping the candle lit in the window for us there. Eve's life has had its own narrative arc and she certainly has her own stories to tell one day.

To my precious mother, Lyn Wellons, who died in 2016—two decades after my father. I am only now beginning to understand the complexities of your life and profound influence on me, in particular on love and all things spiritual. I don't have the words to say how thankful I am for your impact on my life. I am hoping to find them one day soon.

Finally, to my father, John Wellons. I've missed you in these days of later life as I've walked this path that you set me on years ago. But I now know that you've been with me in some way. A large part of this book is about how my patients over the years have helped me come to terms with what a profound influence you were on my life early on, only to lose you and then find you again in my life lived out so far. A cycle of discovery I would wish for anyone—from joy to grief to joy again.

Index

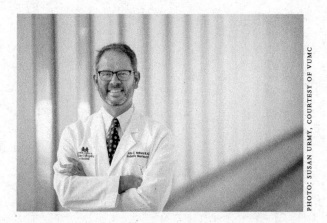

JAY WELLONS, MD, MSPH, is a professor in the departments of neurological surgery, pediatrics, plastic surgery, radiology, and radiological sciences at the Monroe Carell Jr. Children's Hospital at Vanderbilt and the Vanderbilt University Medical Center. He holds the Cal Turner Chair, is the Chief of the Division of Pediatric Neurosurgery, and is the medical director for the Surgical Outcomes Center for Kids (SOCKs), which he co-founded. He has written op-eds for *The New York Times*. Jay Wellons lives in Nashville, Tennessee, with his family.

ABOUT THE TYPE

This book was set in Dante, a typeface designed by Giovanni Mardersteig (1892–1977). Conceived as a private type for the Officina Bodoni in Verona, Italy, Dante was originally cut only for hand composition by Charles Malin, the famous Parisian punch cutter, between 1946 and 1952. Its first use was in an edition of Boccaccio's *Trattatello in laude di Dante* that appeared in 1954. The Monotype Corporation's version of Dante followed in 1957. Though modeled on the Aldine type used for Pietro Cardinal Bembo's treatise *De Aetna* in 1495, Dante is a thoroughly modern interpretation of that venerable face.